ROOT CAUSES

ROOT CAUSES

*Why the Healthcare System is Failing Us
and What We Can Do About It*

DR. AVERY R. CHAMPAGNE

PALMETTO

P U B L I S H I N G

Charleston, SC
www.PalmettoPublishing.com

Copyright © 2025 by Dr. Avery R. Champagne

Paperback ISBN: 9798822973688

For Joyce

CONTENTS

INTRODUCTION

T HIS BOOK IS about *modern health care*—globally, with a primary focus on the United States—and *root causes*, especially the *root cause* of our medical dependency and all the adverse societal effects this dependency has caused. But let's start with some historical perspective to ground ourselves with facts and understandings, and a humble man who became a true hero.

Sakichi Toyoda was born on Valentine's Day 1867 in Yamaguchi-Mura, Tōtōmi Province, about 230 km south of Tokyo. His father, Ikichi, was a farmer, like most men in the region, but also a carpenter. His mother, Ei, was said to be loving and industrious. Like all the other families living in this region of Japan, they lived in poverty.

Sakichi was born during an auspicious period for the Japanese people. With the fall of Japan's military government, the Tokugawa shogunate, a political revolution was underway, and power was being restored to imperial rule. This revolution, better known as the Meiji Restoration, brought about great change in Japan. These were the early years of what we know as modern Japan, and as with any great revolution, social upheaval followed.

When Sakichi graduated from elementary school, he began apprenticing in his father's carpentry business. He was always learning, always reading whatever was available: books, newspaper clippings, and magazines. He had a deep desire to learn and share knowledge with his struggling community. On days he wasn't working, Sakichi would encourage his friends and the local youth to get together to read and study. He had also become obsessed with machinery and the possibilities it provided for his community. Sakichi knew there was an unsolved efficiency problem. At the time, steam was the primary catalyst for automation and machinery, but it was coal powered and thus both dirty and terribly expensive.

Sakichi knew there had to be a better way. In 1885, the Patent Monopoly Act was passed, and Sakichi saw the new possibilities for revolutionizing machinery in Japan. In 1890, he traveled to Tokyo to attend the third National Machinery Exposition. He was beginning to believe he had found his way out of poverty.

Sakichi was fascinated by the technology of the farmers' hand loom, a simple machine designed to create fabric by placing tension on the warp threads and interlacing them with the weft threads. This process was elemental to Japanese lifestyle and culture at the time. If you could efficiently produce fabric to sell, you could easily feed your family, send your children to higher education, and prosper. However, handweaving was also laborious and backbreaking. These rudimentary machines were always breaking down or creating defective material.

After much trial and error, Sakichi Toyoda, still only a twenty-four-year-old carpenter with an elementary school education, successfully produced his first patent: the Toyoda wooden hand loom. This invention increased productivity and effectiveness up to 5 percent for his community of farmers. Sakichi's loom required only one hand to operate, whereas all others required both hands. Now fabric was being produced at a greater rate with higher quality. However, it was still a manual process, and so Sakichi's focus turned to automation.

From 1891 to 1896, Sakichi pioneered several cutting-edge inventions that revolutionized Japanese machinery. He started up factories and companies to further the development of his products and to distribute his fabric, amassing more funds for his research and growing his reputation. In 1894, he produced the Toyoda winding machine and, in 1896, Japan's first-ever power loom. Built of steel and wood, it incorporated an automatic stop mechanism known as the *jidoka*. This is where Sakichi Toyoda's legacy really began. The jidoka allowed anyone to stop all production of fabric, identify the issue, resolve it, and then continue production with an increased quality and efficiency. This feature was ahead of its time and embodied the philosophy that made Sakichi Toyoda so great: a dedication to eliminating waste.

Sakichi's family members then helped him establish Toyoda Automatic Loom Works, which in 1933 established a division dedicated to automobile production, headed up by Sakichi's son Kiichiro. Toyota Motor Corporation was registered independently of Toyoda Loom Works in 1937. Sakichi Toyoda to this day influences countless engineers and inventors across the world to excel and think outside the box.

This is not the story of Toyota Motors or its progressive leaders throughout history. Nor is the point of this account to compare different fabric machines or automobiles. The critical message of Toyoda's success and legacy is found in his *philosophical dedication to understanding*. Sakichi Toyoda knew how to think, problem-solve, and identify *causes* and *effects*. He systematized this process, naming it *The 5 Whys*.

Taiichi Ohno, the father of Toyota's production system, acknowledged that the basis of Toyota's scientific approach is to ask *why* five times whenever they find a problem. By doing this, the nature of the problem as well as its solution becomes clear. This system of questioning and identifying issues is so effective in engineering, technology, and leadership that it has been widely adopted as the philosophy behind the productivity systems of Kaizen, Six Sigma, and lean manufacturing.

Let's use this method together to look at an everyday problem. Let's ask ourselves "Why?" five times and see if we can't get to the *root cause* of the issue. Traffic is an easy example. We've all experienced headaches with traffic, such as running late or missing exits. We all make driving mistakes, even illegal ones. Try this method now on this problem: You ran a red light and got a ticket.

1. Why? You were late for work.
2. Why? You woke up late.
3. Why? Your alarm didn't go off.
4. Why? Your phone was dead.
5. Why? You didn't properly plug in the charger before bed (*root cause!*)

Applying Sakichi's methodology, the root cause of your problem was human and process oriented. Many technical problems can be traced back to human factors and process-driven systems.

For any problem you have, any issue you face today, the root cause can and must be identified. Informed decision-making is the only way out of the problems we face, individually or societally. And such is the case for our health care. As stated at the beginning, this book is about *modern health care* and *root causes.*

The health care system in this country has turned into a full-fledged art form for its providers. Our Michelangelos and da Vincis may not be creating a *David* or *The Last Supper*; they are, however, shelling out billions annually on prescription medication advertising and lobbying measures for pharmaceuticals and experimental surgical technology. Think fewer paintbrushes and more black Prada suits driving E-Class Mercedes-Benzes.

Have you ever lain in a hospital bed? We've seen movies in which a man is coming out of a comatose state in a quiet, dimly lit room with hushed voices around him. The reality is far different. That room is incredibly fluorescent and artificial. A symphony of sounds is constantly being emitted from the electronic devices ensuring survival: pumps, medication dispensers, ventilators, fluid warmers, respiratory and EKG/ECG monitors.

Despite the obvious and apparent issues our country faces today on many fronts, you would at the very least expect that this is the *best* place to have a health crisis, right? Where else in the world do we have access to cutting-edge surgical technology, state-of-the-art diagnostic imaging, and superior medical know-how? Never mind *why*—the fact remains that the country that most regularly uses such tools should have the most to show for it…right?

Not necessarily. In 2014, the Department of Health Care Policy at Harvard Medical School funded a study of Medicare beneficiaries that aimed to identify commonly used tests and procedures and identify whether they were considered *low-value.* When medical agencies or research organizations consistently find no added benefit to a patient's health or outcome, they deem the procedure, drug, or test as low-value. After an entire year of carefully researching the literature, analyzing our common medical practices, and including 1,360,908 Medicare patients, it was clear that anywhere from 25 percent to 42 percent of those patients received *at least* one low-value service.[1]

Think of all the people you know who are on Medicare or are eligible for it. How does it feel to know that as you read these words, they are being overexamined and overtreated with *no added benefit* to their health? What if some of these interventions pushed on your friends and family even caused harm? Why are many of us comfortable with these facts? Is there a root cause (or root causes) for this sad state of affairs?

Let's start with the here and now: the state of our health care. By most metrics, we, the United States, are one of the most medicated and pro-surgery countries in the world. Almost 66 percent of the US population is actively taking prescribed medication—antihypertensives, pain relievers, and especially mental health drugs.[2] What does our current relationship with traditional health care give us? The most Olympic athletes? Longest life spans? What about the lowest infant mortality rates? Unfortunately, the answer to all three is a resounding "No."

---

[1]   Aaron L. Schwartz et al., "Measuring Low-Value Care in Medicare," *JAMA Internal Medicine* 174, no. 7 (2014): 1067–1076.

[2]   Robin Osborn, David Squires, and Michelle M. Doty, "Paying for Prescription Drugs Around the World: Why Is the U.S. an Outlier?" *The Commonwealth Fund*, October 16, 2017, https://www.commonwealthfund.org/publications/issue-briefs/2017/oct/paying-prescription-drugs-around-world-why-us-outlier.

Six out of ten Americans are living with a chronic condition such as heart disease or cancer. This is the alarming reality being recorded by the CDC, the WHO, and countless others right now. The level of heart disease has become so critical that it is claiming the lives of 877,500 Americans every year.[3] Wouldn't you think that, given this reality, we would at the least know how to deal with it effectively and efficiently? The Mayo Clinic defines coronary heart disease (CAD) as "damage or disease in the heart's major blood vessels." The usual suspect is plaque buildup that causes coronary arteries to narrow, limiting blood flow to the heart. Symptoms range from none to chest pain (angina), shortness of breath, and heart attack.

One of the most common ways of dealing with CAD is by inserting a stent, a metal tube that slips into the artery and forces it open. This procedure occurs *four hundred thousand times a year*. It should be noted that the procedure is used to treat *stable* coronary artery disease, meaning symptoms are not getting worse, they last for short amounts of time, and they subside with rest.[4]

---

[3] "Heart Disease and Stroke Prevention: Factsheet," Centers for Disease Control and Prevention, https://www.cdc.gov/chronicdisease/resources/publications/factsheets/heart-disease-stroke.htm.

[4] Mitchell H. Katz and Vinay Prasad, "The Surprising History of the 'NNT,'" *JAMA Internal Medicine* 171, no. 13 (2011): 1272–1274.

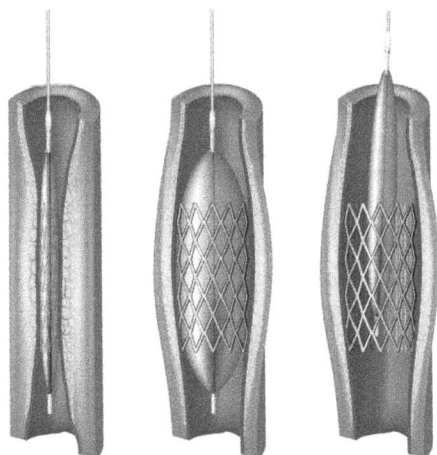

Illustration of an arterial stent.

Surely a procedure that is so commonplace in our country has a fantastic track record and has results in no way similar to those of the Medicare study previously mentioned. Well, a 2012 meta-analysis examined *every randomized clinical trial* that compared stent implantation with more conservative forms of treatment, such as exercise and lifestyle changes, and there was *no evidence of benefit* in the form of prevention of death and heart attack compared with initial medical therapy such as conservative medication and major lifestyle changes.[5]

No evidence of benefiting a patient's quality of life, yet four hundred thousand people will still be advised to undergo this procedure.

There is a significant problem here, and its roots run deep. Already you may be drawing conclusions, perhaps experiencing

---

[5] Nikolas J. Stergiopoulos and David L. Brown, "Initial Coronary Stent Implantation with Medical Therapy vs Medical Therapy Alone for Stable Coronary Artery Disease," *Archives of Internal Medicine* 172, no. 4 (2012): 312–19, https://doi.org/10.1001/archinternmed.2011.1484..

feelings of frustration and resentment toward medical institutions and professionals. How can a country like the United States, with an urgent care clinic on every corner and medications available for every ailment, be so sick and diseased? How can we be home to some of the most prestigious universities in the world, such as Harvard Medical School and Johns Hopkins, and still be so blind to data such as this? If you have these feelings, you are not being irrational.

On the other hand, reading this might make you feel defensive and annoyed. Perhaps you're in the medical field yourself or you love a medical professional who has sacrificed countless hours to fight for others' survival. But this is not an attack on medical professionals—this problem unfortunately encompasses them as well.

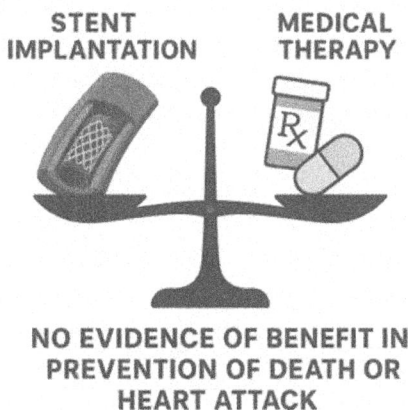

STENT IMPLANTATION   **MEDICAL THERAPY**

NO EVIDENCE OF BENEFIT IN PREVENTION OF DEATH OR HEART ATTACK

*

So what about the medical professionals? They are the heroes fighting on the front lines every day and working their hardest to ensure survival, and they are under immense pressure. The system as it's currently being used is bursting at the seams. Our nurses and doctors are overworked, under tremendous stress, and underappreciated. We've all heard the term *burnout,* first coined in the early 1970s by psychoanalyst Herbert Freudenberger and later used to describe the physiological toll it takes. Burnout involves "emotional exhaustion, cynicism and depersonalization, reduced professional efficacy and personal accomplishment." And when it comes to our health care workers, it's abundantly clear that their mental and physical well-being are not being protected. If they are the heroes our media personalities and politicians claim they are, how can we allow their well-being to slip so far? Burnout is a growing health phenomenon that needs to be better understood and dealt with. This term is *not* limited to the health care profession; whatever your profession, you might be experiencing these feelings yourself. However, it is disproportionately affecting health care workers.

Recent studies have shown that over 50 percent of all physicians in the United States are experiencing burnout.[6] And it's only getting worse. A 2013 survey asked 20,000 US attending physicians about their lifestyles. At that time, the burnout rate was 45.8 percent. The same organization in 2017 surveyed over 14,000 US physicians across more than 30 specialties. This report revealed that the overall physician burnout rate had increased to 51 percent, marking a significant rise from previous years. Notably, certain specialties reported even higher rates, with emergency medicine physicians experiencing a 59 percent burnout rate.[7]

[6] Tait D. Shanafelt et al., "Burnout and Satisfaction with Work-Life Balance Among US Physicians Relative to the General US Population," *Archives of Internal Medicine* 172 (2012): 1377–1385.

[7] *Medscape Lifestyle Report 2017: Race and Ethnicity, Bias and Burnout,* https://www.medscape.com/features/slideshow/lifestyle/2017/overview.

If you've ever found yourself in a hospital or emergency room, or supporting a family member in those situations, you probably have a profound admiration for the nursing staff. Nurses are perhaps the most overused and underappreciated health care workers in our country. Nurses are constantly on the go—conducting physical exams, taking vitals, recording histories, monitoring conditions, drawing blood, cleaning patients, providing education and emotional support—the list goes on and on. Is there an association between our jam-packed hospitals and the health of our nurses?

A 2001 study found that a staggering 43 percent of nurses working at US hospitals experience symptoms of emotional and physical exhaustion.[8] For a career that depends heavily on quick thinking, fast problem-solving, and clear-headed decisiveness, it's likely that a nurse's emotional and physical health massively affects health outcomes. In 2017, registered nurses had 24,540 reported incidents of illness or injury resulting in one or more days away from work. Nursing assistants reported an additional 34,210 incidents in the same year—an incidence rate exceeded only by law enforcement patrol officers.[9] According to a study in the *Journal of the American Medical Association*, each additional patient over four, per nurse, carries a 23 percent risk of increased burnout and a 15 percent decrease in job satisfaction. The same study found that each additional patient per nurse

---

[8] Linda H. Aiken et al., "Nurses' Reports on Hospital Care in Five Countries," *Health Affairs* 20, no. 3 (2001): 43–53.

[9] Department for Professional Employees, AFL-CIO, "Safe Staffing Critical for Patients and Nurses," https://www.dpeaflcio.org/factsheets/safe-staffing-critical-for-patients-and-nurses.

was associated with a 7 percent increase in the likelihood of a patient dying within thirty days of admission.[10]

Does this problem start to look somewhat self-reinforcing to you yet?

Even the health of our medical students is becoming affected. The average age of a medical student is early to mid-twenties, an age group usually associated with vigor, energy, and strong physical health. A 2013 review estimated that *at least half* of students at US medical schools experience symptoms of burnout, and a 2018 meta-analysis of over 16,000 students worldwide found that 44 percent suffered from burnout.[11]

Our health care system is the problem. All of it. Our quality of health. The toll health care has on its workers. The outcomes we are getting. *The actual lack of health in our society.*

But before we get too buried in heavy statistics and heart-breaking accounts of families and health disparities, let's pause. We'll return to this. Right now, there is a more urgent question to be asked—one that addresses the unconscious and emotional connotation we've attached to the entire health care industry: *How* did we become so *dependent* on traditional medicine?

---

[10]   Linda H. Aiken et al., "Hospital Nurse Staffing and Patient Mortality, Nurse Burnout, and Job Dissatisfaction," *JAMA* 288, no. 16 (2002): 1987–1993.

[11]   W. IsHak et al., "Burnout in Medical Students: A Systematic Review," *The Clinical Teacher* 10 (2013): 242–245; Lionel Frajerman et al., "Burnout in Medical Students: A Systematic Review and Meta-Analysis," *European Psychiatry* 55 (2019): 36–42.

What is the root cause?

Every facet of American culture involves medical dependency in some form or another. Turn on the television. You won't go more than sixty seconds before you hear the infamous line, "Ask your doctor if…" Go to a standard urgent care or ER. They are packed full. Medical dependency is such an issue that we now have independent doctors urging people *not* to diagnose themselves on popular sites such as WebMD.

Using our newfound root cause analysis skills, can we look deeper? Instead of pointing the finger and assigning blame over the problems we face, can we instead understand how this medical dependency came to be?

- How far back has our society relied on the traditional medical system?
- What's feeding into that dependency today?
- What are we getting as a society by using the traditional health care system as it exists today?
- And finally…
- Is there anything to be gained by embracing new and updated health practices?

Within answers to these questions lies the *root cause* of our problems with the *traditional* health care industry. As Sakichi Toyoda had done thousands of times before, it is time we identify the *root cause* if we are ever going to create a healthier and improved future for ourselves. A future in which…

Six out of ten Americans *do not* live with a chronic disease.

We don't spend over 3 trillion dollars a year on health care expenses.

Politicians and industries don't benefit from our illnesses.

Children grow up in families not burdened by health care debt.

People are empowered to take their health into their own hands.

My hope is that by the end of this exploration of history and modern society, we can make some much-needed empowered choices for our health. But it must start with us and our choice to deviate from societal norms and disengage from those deeply rooted practices they still uphold.

CHAPTER 1

SPIRITUAL ROOTS

"Make a habit of two things: to help, or at least to do no harm."

—Hippocrates

I F WE WANT to understand where our enormous dependency on modern-day traditional medicine stems from, we must first appreciate the environment in which healers originated and the spiritual role they served. Much of the healing art practiced in the ancient civilizations has been intimately married to spirituality and religion—the societal glue that held all of these great civilizations together. Many of these institutions remain powerful to this day.

But we live in a time when survival is no longer tribal. We can venture far from our place of birth and be just fine. The strength of our family unit, tribe, or village is not the determining factor for how well we fare in this world. This was not the case just a few hundred years ago. Where you came from mattered, and who you lived with and around was in many ways a matter of life or death. Religion and spiritual practices were essential in maintaining familial bonds, the strength of one's tribe, and the cohesiveness of a village or region. You do not have to look very closely into any civilization's history (ancient or modern) to see the instrumentality of spirituality or religion.

Religion has perhaps been the biggest catalyst for change in the modern history of the world, whether it be sparking wars; shaping politics and geography; or spreading language, science, and art—and yes, disease, illness, and violence. But this is not a critique or a dissection of the powerful force that exists in this world, only a reminder that everything of importance in the ancient days of civilization and society was intimately conjoined with spirituality and religion. Which brings us to the healers.

There are many names for healers of all kinds throughout the centuries: shaman, medicine man or woman, witch doctor, apothecary, and so on. People living in America before the arrival of Europeans referred to their healers as medicine men or women. Even the smallest bit of research into the healing practices of Native Americans can show just how expansive and diverse their understanding of spirituality, religion, and healing approaches were, and continue to be. There are now over five hundred federally recognized Native tribes in the United States and many more tribal subsets. Though all have their own unique beliefs, there are some commonalities worth noting.

Indigenous medicine men and women were not mechanistic in their view of the body. Their practices were not *allopathic* (based on current scientific evidence and prescription of conventional treatments) or single-minded. Every action taken to help diagnose, treat, or cure an individual was based on their connection to spirit. One of their most unifying beliefs is that all things in nature are connected. Sicangu-Oglala Lakota Chief Luther Standing Bear once wrote:

"The Earth was full of sounds which the old-time Indian could hear, sometimes putting his ear to it so as to hear more clearly. The forefathers of the Lakotas had done this for long ages until there had come to them a real understanding of Earth ways. It was almost as if the man were still part of the Earth as he was in the beginning."[12]

Many of the healing practices used by Native healers were to establish connection with nature, asking for guidance by spirit, or in some instances, warding off spirits that might be causing ill health or misfortune. Even the word *medicine* has different meanings depending on the context. When we hear that word today, we imagine a pill or liquid taken to treat a specific illness. With many Native Americans, the word could refer to a collection of sacred tokens. Pretty-Shield, a medicine woman of the Crow, remembered her father's medicine as he rode off to battle: "He gave the Crow war cry, and then, armed only with his medicine, the stuffed skin of the long-legged owl, tied on his head, and his coup stick, he rode out alone against his enemy."[13]

Many medicine men and women were also priests and authority figures on all things spiritual. Prominent Native American activist and theologian Vine Deloria Jr., when writing about the powers of medicine men, thought a more accurate description would be "holy ones, people who have lived a more vigorous and disciplined life."[14]

---

[12] Standing Bear, Luther. *Land of the Spotted Eagle*. Lincoln and London: University of Nebraska Press.

[13] Frank B. Linderman, *Pretty-Shield: Medicine Woman of the Crows* (New York: HarperCollins, 2021).

[14] Vine Deloria Jr., *The World We Used to Live In: Remembering the Powers of the Medicine Men* (Golden, CO: Fulcrum Publishing, 2006), xxv–xxvi.

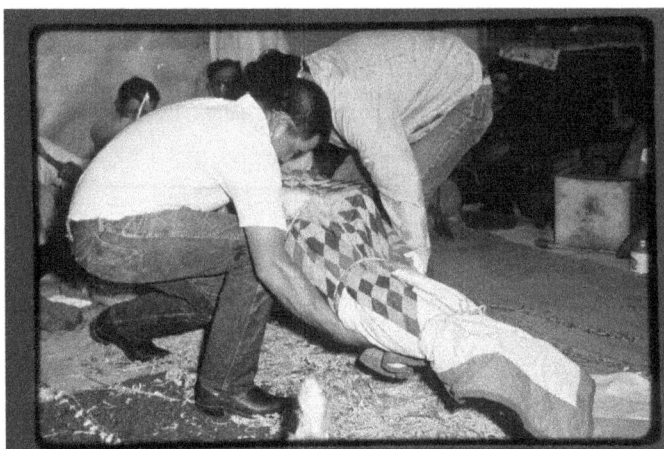

Photograph of a Yuwipi Ceremony in action.
Captured by Richard Erdoes.

Or consider the Yuwipi ceremony. Traditionally used by the Lakota and other Plains tribes, the ceremony involved a medicine vision, or dream, giving the medicine man, as the main facilitator, the opportunity to receive sacred communication with spirits regarding problems, the future, or healing crises. Before the ceremony, he would instruct others to bind his arms and legs together, wrap him entirely in buffalo robes, and place him in the middle of a tipi or lodge that was sealed from all light. He was surrounded by four hundred or more offerings of tobacco for any spirits who might enter and participate in the healing ceremony. Once the process began, the medicine man sang the sacred songs and did not stop until the ceremony was completed when the sick people were healed or the future was predicted. It should be noted that the Yuwipi ceremony was a rather large undertaking, with many participants both observing and facilitating, and did not take place very often.

There were, however, everyday practices that the medicine man was also responsible for. One of Native America's most enduring and well-known healing practices is plant medicine, from which over two hundred herbs and plants are still used in pharmaceutical form today, such as willow bark. Indigenous North Americans would chew on willow bark or boil its leaves and drink the tea to relieve a whole host of health problems, from headaches to joint pain and even dental caries and abscesses. Willow bark contains acetylsalicylic acid, the primary ingredient in aspirin.[15]

Aztec and Mayan people also used this approach when it came to health interventions. If someone under their care fell ill, they knew there had to be an imbalance in the mind/body/spirit connection. Whether it was Aztec forms of *pulque* or *octili* (fermented aloe) to dull pains and injuries, ground volcanic obsidian to rub into ulcers and rashes, or herbs used by Mayans to induce vomiting and bowel movements, the intentions were always focused on spirit—restoring connection to the spirit world or warding off the spirits that could be causing the sickness. The Mayans also had their own class of revered healers, called *ah'men*. Ah'men had many responsibilities, ranging from diagnosing and treating conditions to therapy and counseling, and even administering hallucinogenic plants to help bring the sick closer to the gods.

The full extent of the indigenous Americans' knowledge of healing, spirituality, and nature may never be fully known to the "outside world." But when we take a step back to appreciate the different cultures and societies that first populated America and continue in some form today, a few things are clear. *Humans did not exist independently from nature.* Plants, animals, and spirits played perhaps the largest role in the healing process. *Spirituality* was woven into every fabric of the lifestyle, which is why it should be no surprise to see how elemental medicine

---

[15] Steve Parker, *A Short History of Medicine* (New York: DK, 2019).

men and women were in their tribes. Whether those healers asked for it or not, they were authority figures. Helping people navigate the spiritual realm, seek out answers, live longer, and rid themselves of illnesses was sacred work that continues today. Salish author Mourning Dove (1884–1936) said it perfectly: "Everything on the earth has a purpose, every disease an herb to cure it, and every person a mission. This is the Indian theory of existence."[16]

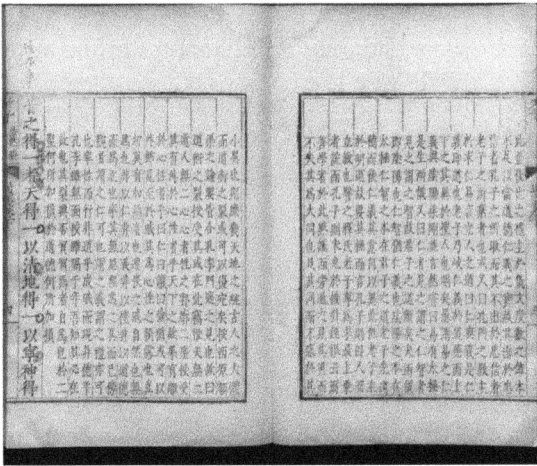

The Tao Te Ching is widely considered one of the foundational texts of Taoism and one of the most influential works in Chinese philosophy and world literature.

As beautiful as the origins of healing are in the Americas, there are similar origin stories for healing that can be found elsewhere in the world. The concepts of balance, energy, and nature were just as essential in ancient China. Any endeavor to understand the basics of how Chinese people approached health must start with their own philosophy, just as it would have been

---

[16]   Mourning Dove, quoted in "Mourning Dove," *Encyclopedia of World Biography*, 2nd ed., vol. 9 (Gale, 2004), 222.

confusing to study the intricate Yuwipi ceremony without an understanding of the Lakota views of health and spirituality. The dominating Chinese philosophy for the past two millennia has been Taoism. Birthed from scripture written between 770 and 476 BCE, the *Tao Te Ching* is full of poetic and philosophical teachings on the origin of the universe, life and death, and nature, and it even details ways of living with one another. The *Tao Te Ching* is perhaps the earliest philosophical work in Chinese history. Taoism permeates every facet of Chinese society, culture, and governance up to the present day.

Taoism and its principles are so influential that it has even reached modern American culture and society. *Yin* and *yang*, and even the concept of *qi*, are just a few of the essential aspects of Taoism that many Westerners know of. One of the most common themes found within Taoism (or Daoism) is *balance*—harmony in nature.[17] Yin and yang are among the most iconic and well-known symbols in history. This black-and-white figure represents many concepts in life: duality, opposing forces, feminine/masculine, and good/bad. Yin is most often associated with darkness, water, coolness, and the feminine. Yang is associated with brightness, dryness, heat, activity, and the masculine. The *Tao Te Ching* tells us that these two forces are actually complementary and can be found throughout all of life. In Chapter 42, for example, it is written that "the created universe carries the yin at its back and the yang in front; through the union of pervading principles, it reaches harmony".[18] The concepts of nature and order also dominate Tao philosophy. Chapter 25 of the *Tao Te Ching* lays out the natural hierarchy of the universe:

---

[17]   Lin Yutang, *The Wisdom of Laotse* (New York: Modern Library, 1948).

[18]   Lin Yutang, *The Wisdom of Laotse* (New York: Modern Library, 1948).

"Tao is Great,
Tao, the Great!
It is greater than Heaven,
Greater than the Earth.
Greater than the king.
These are the four great things, and the
ruler is the least of them.
Humanity is schooled by the Earth;
Earth is taught by Heaven,
and Heaven is guided by the Tao.
And the Tao goes with what is absolutely natural."[19]

If Tao is "the way" and the Tao does not go against what is naturally occurring, then people should not go against nature, for the natural existence is a state without competition and struggle. Chapter 81 points out:

"A small country has fewer people. Though there are machines that can work ten to a hundred times faster than man, they are not needed. The people take death seriously and do not travel far. Though they have boats and carriages, no one uses them. Though they have armor and weapons, no one displays them. Men return to the knotting of rope in place of writing. Their food is plain and good, their clothes fine but simple, their homes secure; They are happy in their ways."[20]

If you have ever taken a Tai chi class or received acupuncture, you have probably heard of qi, pronounced "chee." The concept of qi is found throughout all eighty-one chapters of the *Tao Te Ching*, where it is often referred to as vital life force

[19] Michael LaFargue, *The Tao of the Tao Te Ching: A Translation and Commentary* (Albany: State University of New York Press, 1992).

[20] Michael LaFargue, *The Tao of the Tao Te Ching: A Translation and Commentary* (Albany: State University of New York Press, 1992).

or vital energy. Qi does not have one universally understood definition. However, the word often refers to the vital life force gained by breathing. It can be our breath itself. Everything that occurs in our life, positive and negative, is because of qi.

Sadly, all of these sacred concepts are often abused, misunderstood, or even appropriated, yet they remain the guiding principles found in traditional Chinese medicine. China and its people have been meticulously documenting health and healing practices for centuries, long before their first unified dynasty and emperor, Qin Shi Huang (259–210 BC). It is quite remarkable how well-preserved their traditions and written history have remained. About 2,000 years ago, between 403 and 221 BCE, one of the first pieces, and certainly the most iconic piece, of Chinese literature on medicine was published: the *Huang-di Nei'Jing*. Translated as *The Yellow Emperor's Classic of Internal Medicine* and composed of two separate texts, *Suwen* and *Lingshu*, these 162 chapters are laid out as a dialogue between the mythical Yellow Emperor, Huang-di, and his advisers or ministers. As with any ancient and influential published works, their original content has been revised many times over. As language evolves and context changes, words can lose their original meaning. Luckily for us, China is well known for meticulous record-keeping and documentation.

The Yellow Emperor's Classic contains extensive methods of diagnosing conditions, classifications of ailments, various treatments, and ways of observing different bodily functions (e.g., pulse, respiration, bowel movements, and urinary health). When one analyzes the first several chapters of this ancient medical encyclopedia, the influence of Taoism is undeniable. Recall the Taoist outlook on yin and yang—to live in accordance with yin and yang is to live in a natural state of harmony.

That is the way of the Tao. Conversations in the very first chapter of *The Yellow Emperor's Classics* outline the health effects of living with balance.

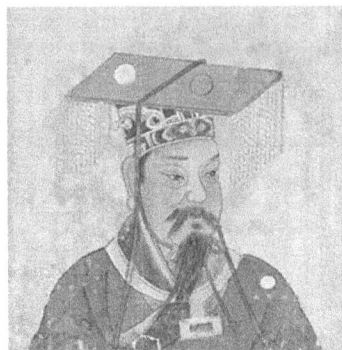

Huangdi, also known as the Yellow Emperor, is considered one of the mythical founding fathers of Chinese civilization.

"The people of high antiquity—those who knew the Way—modeled their behavior on yin and yang and they complied with the arts and the calculations. Their eating and drinking were moderate. Their rising and resting had regularity. They did not tax themselves with meaningless work. Hence, they were able to keep physical appearance and spirit together, and to exhaust the years allotted by heaven.".[21]

The chapter doubles down on the critical role that yin/ yang balance plays in our health:

"Now, the yin and yang [qi] of the four seasons, they constitute root and basis of the myriad beings. Hence, the sages in spring and summer nourish the yang and in autumn and winter nourish the yin, and this way they follow their roots.

---

[21]   Paul U. Unschuld, Hermann Tessenow, and Zheng Jinsheng, *Huang Di Nei Jing Su Wen: An Annotated Translation of Huang Di's Inner Classic* (University of California Press, 2011), 1–4.

Hence, they are in the depth or at the surface with the myriad beings at the gate to life and growth. To oppose one's root, is to attack one's basis and to spoil one's true [qi]. Hence, yin [qi], yang [qi], and the four seasons, they constitute end and begin of the myriad beings, they are the basis of death and life. Opposing them results in catastrophe and harms life. If one follows them, severe diseases will not emerge. This is called 'to achieve the Way'."[22]

Chapter 4 goes into further detail on the *anatomy and physiology* of the human body and how it relates to yin and yang. The five visceral organs (heart, lungs, liver, kidneys, and spleen) are all yin. The stomach, intestines, gallbladder, and urinary bladder are yang. Further mirroring Taoist themes of nature and harmony, *The Yellow Emperor's Classic* details the five phases (wood, earth, water, fire, and metal) and how each phase influences each organ. Each season (spring, summer, autumn, and winter) has different influences on the yin and yang within the body.

According to *The Yellow Emperor's Classic*, "a good diagnostician will observe the patient's complexion, take his pulse, and take the first step of determining whether it is a Yin disease or a Yang disease."[23] The treating physician will examine the pulse, respiration, and complexion in a myriad of ways to determine the organ in question, the nature of the disease, and what seasonal and elemental influences are in play. It is the careful and humble

---

[22] Paul U. Unschuld, Hermann Tessenow, and Zheng Jinsheng, *Huang Di Nei Jing Su Wen: An Annotated Translation of Huang Di's Inner Classic* (University of California Press, 2011), 1–4.

[23] Paul U. Unschuld, Hermann Tessenow, and Zheng Jinsheng, *Huang Di Nei Jing Su Wen: An Annotated Translation of Huang Di's Inner Classic* (University of California Press, 2011), 1–4.

diagnosis that will dictate the minimal intervention. The intervention, as outlined in *The Yellow Emperor's Classic*, depends on the organ in question, where in the disease process the patient is, which energies are involved, the current season, and whether the disease is a problem of excess or a problem of deficiency. Balance is the way in both Taoist philosophy and Chinese medicine.

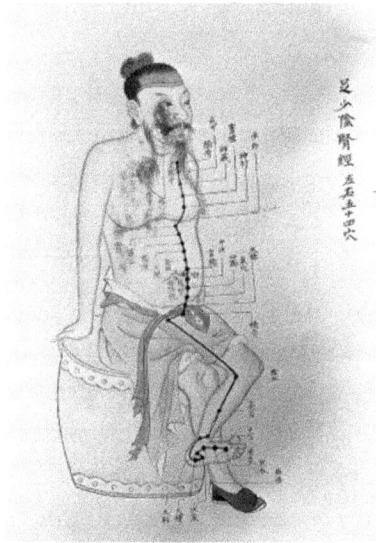

Acupuncture was meticulously documented in ancient Chinese medicine, particularly in the Huangdi Neijing, which outlines meridian pathways, point locations, and therapeutic techniques that form the foundation of traditional Chinese medical practice.

As scientific understanding evolves, so too have Chinese practices. Yet one of the most unchanged healing practices throughout Chinese history is the art of acupuncture. Traditional Chinese medicine saw disease and illness as a disturbance in the flow of qi, whether it be from yin organ disturbances affecting yang or yang acting on yin. Ancient acupuncturists sought to free up qi and restore harmony to the flow of life force. They did this by accessing the body channels referred to in *The Yellow Emperor's Classic* as *meridian points*.

Vital life force, or qi, is not an abstract concept for Chinese healers. Nature, the elements, seasons—all have a direct effect on the expression of qi, and the healers know the consequences of having balance thrown off. Here is just one small example of the recorded physiological effects of qi and meridians in Chapter 3 of *The Yellow Emperor's Classic*: "When cold energy invades the body and causes a depression to the meridians, running sores may come about as a result of its residing in between the muscles and pores. If the energy of meridians becomes thin and deficient, the cold energy may pass through it to attack the viscera and bowels and cause fear and shock."[24]

Acupuncturists have to locate the source of imbalance through meticulous diagnosis. They often observe pulse, respiration, the tongue, and the color of the eyes, urine, and feces. Once determined, they then choose the different access points on the patient's body. These points of access, or *acupuncture points*, often overlap with meridians in the body. The *Huang-di Nei'Jing* details over three hundred different acupuncture points in the body. By inserting a sharp, thin needle into the skin, the practitioner can then redirect the flow of qi through the appropriate meridians. Every meridian channel in the body was specifically linked to anatomy and physiology. This is best exemplified in Chapter 4 of *The Yellow Emperor's Classic*: "Energy of the liver meridian enters into the neck; the energy of the heart meridian enters into the chest and the ribs; the energy of the lungs' meridian enters into the shoulder and the

---

[24] Paul U. Unschuld, Hermann Tessenow, and Zheng Jinsheng, *Huang Di Nei Jing Su Wen: An Annotated Translation of Huang Di's Inner Classic* (University of California Press, 2011), 1–4.

back; the energy of the kidney's meridian enters into the loins and the thigh…. The energy of the spleen meridian enters into the spine." [25]

This ancient and revered approach to health has been well maintained throughout thousands of years. Thankfully, these methods of healing have reached the West and established strong footholds. Acupuncture and the holistic view of the mind and body still play an integral role in medicine. Acupuncture is widely available across the world. How amazing is the legacy of *The Huang-di Nei'Jing*? Though written thousands of years ago, it has influenced millions of physicians across the globe and shaped the health care of one of the oldest and longest-standing nations in the world. Without Taoism, there would be no *Huang-di Nei'Jing*. They go hand in hand. This is one of China's greatest strengths, its enduring legacy. Taoist philosophy still permeates every aspect of the Chinese lifestyle. To diverge from this is to question the way of life.

This idea that we are chasing, that spirituality and religion were intertwined with the healing practices of earlier times, can be well exemplified by the pharaohs and priests of ancient Egypt. In fact, the entire region incorporated spirituality and religion into everyday practices. Many of us have seen hieroglyphics depicting humans with the heads of animals, embalming of the dead, and construction projects that have stood the test of time built to appease the gods and their kings (whom they thought of as gods).

The earliest forms of writing from Mesopotamia (present-day Iraq, Turkey, and Syria) detail specific ancient practices.

---

[25] Paul U. Unschuld, Hermann Tessenow, and Zheng Jinsheng, *Huang Di Nei Jing Su Wen: An Annotated Translation of Huang Di's Inner Classic* (University of California Press, 2011), 1–4.

Medical authorities known as *ashipus* declared that illnesses, disease, and injury could be attributed to evil spirits, and only the ashipus could determine which evil spirit was the source of an ailment. Through means of sorcery, chants, spells, or even curses, they drove them out, restoring the health of an individual. There were also the *asus*. Distinctly different from but often working in collaboration with the ashipus, the asus were less concerned with magic and spells and more dedicated to the hands-on healing approach: preparing herbal tinctures, sanitizing and wrapping wounds, rubbing oils onto injuries, and massage. Both of these classes of healers were important, but it should be noted that the ashipus were often held in higher regard because of their spiritual authority.[26]

Egyptian novelist Naguib Mahfouz once wrote, "If you want to move people, you look for a point of sensitivity, and in Egypt, nothing moves people as much as religion."[27] This could easily be said about most of the great early civilizations. The kingdoms in the Middle East made great advances in art, science, math, and chemistry, but religion reigned supreme over all of these. How fascinating it is that while ancient Egyptian texts were carefully documenting injuries on the brain and cervical spine (neck) and even mentioning cerebrospinal fluid, ancient Egyptians were praying to the scorpion goddess Serket when they were bitten by a scorpion.[28]

Priests and doctors were often one and the same. Bringing forth godly protection was often necessary because disease, injury, and natural disaster were just a part of everyday life. Many healers were priests of Sekhmet (the goddess of healing,

---

26   Steve Parker, *A Short History of Medicine* (New York: DK, 2019).

27   C. Shabrawy, interview with Naguib Mahfouz, 1992.

28   Steve Parker, *A Short History of Medicine* (New York: DK, 2019).

curses, and threats), and so daily healing practices involved the use of amulets, aromas, offerings, and incantations, all to call forth and please the gods, or a particular god. More practical treatment methods were widely used as well.

Similar to the ashipus and asus in Mesopotamia, there were distinct differences between Egyptian priests and more traditional physicians and their scribes, who heavily documented their findings and observations on papyrus scrolls. A few of these scrolls have survived, containing religious texts, journalistic accountings of construction projects, and, of course, medical records. One of the best known is referred to as the *Edwin Smith Papyrus*. Named after an American Egyptologist, it dates back 3,600 years. Unlike other writings of the times, the *Smith Papyrus* does not contain extensive spells and incantations, but it does go into great detail on anatomical understanding and brain and spinal injuries. It also details various surgeries and their tools. The format is extremely organized, starting with the head and working its way down to the lower back. There are forty-eight case histories in the scroll, and it is surprisingly thorough in its approach to examination, observations, prognosis, and treatment methods.

A common philosophy was adopted throughout ancient Egypt when it came to practicing medicine (religious or practical). After a physician was done assessing a patient, the physician then assigned him or her to one of three categories:

Treatable injuries were handled immediately.

Contestable injuries were considered to not be life-threatening. The patient was expected to survive without intervention by the doctor, so patients were simply observed.

Untreatable ailments were not subjected to any intervention by doctors.

Another noteworthy papyrus scroll pertaining to health is the *Ebers Papyrus*. This impressive record can be dated back to 3,500 years ago. It is about a foot tall and twenty meters long. Unlike the *Smith Papyrus*, the *Ebers Papyrus* contains magical spells, incantations, and herbal remedies, well over seven hundred of them.[29] Though it was far less organized and systematic than the *Smith Papyrus*, it did contain much useful information, such as the following treatments for certain conditions:

Asthma: honey and milk, sesame, frankincense

Headaches: poppy seeds, aloe

Burns and skin diseases: aloe

Pain relief: thyme

Digestive aids: juniper, mint, garlic, sandalwood

Chest pains: mustard seeds, aloe, juniper

Dressing a wound: honey (which is a natural antibiotic).[30]

To preserve the papyrus scrolls as best they could, the Egyptians kept them in the part of their temples known as the Per-Ankh, or the House of Life. It was here also that scribes, priests, and physicians would study their craft, lecture, and transcribe their knowledge.

---

[29] Kara Rogers, *Medicine and Healers Through History* (New York: The Rosen Publishing Group, 2011).

[30] *The Papyrus Ebers*, trans. Cyrill Phillips Bryan (London: Ares Publishers Inc., 1930).

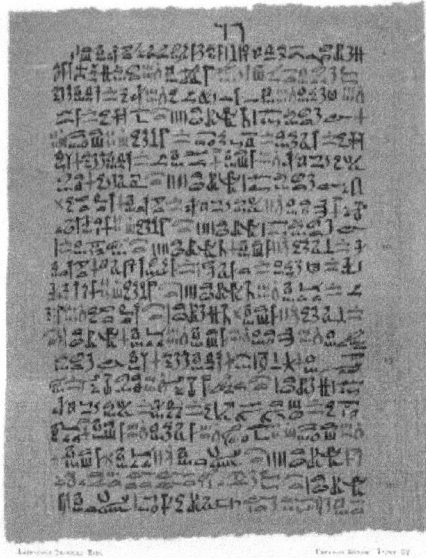

Prescription treatment for asthma found
in the ancient Ebers papyrus.

Here's the thing. It's fun analyzing the various healing
techniques and cultures throughout history and admiring and
appreciating how their views on spirituality and nature affected
their everyday life, including medicine. But the reason we are
spending so much time dissecting these ancient belief patterns
is to highlight the incredibly strong reverence our society still
places on such institutions. Science and understanding have
certainly evolved throughout the millennia, but our feelings
toward these powerful institutions have not. At least not in a
substantial way. Want to know just how influential ancient
Egyptian medicine still is in our world?

Consider the Egyptian god of magic, Heka. He represents
the vital force that powers magic and healing, illustrating how
deeply magic was woven into Egyptian society. The Greeks developed their own healing traditions, symbolized by the **Rod of**

Asclepius, a staff with a single entwined serpent, which became a lasting symbol of medicine. While the modern medical profession often uses the **caduceus**—a staff with two intertwined serpents—this symbol is historically linked to Hermes, the Greek god of commerce and communication, rather than healing. Today anyone in a medical emergency seeing that iconic symbol will be comforted, knowing that they are in the right place, resonating with five thousand years of societal influence. Medicine, surgery, and healing in general have always served a crucial role in every community. Modern medicine may not be associated with spells and spirits, but it's hard to deny that healers throughout history and into the present have been elevated to a higher class of authority. And maybe rightly so; it's clear that to become a skilled and respected healer, one must prove oneself to be of high intellect, discipline, and compassion—important attributes of any leader.

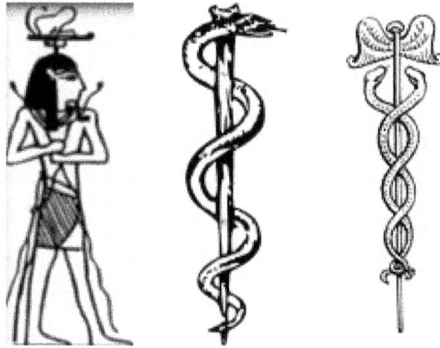

From left to right: Heka holding two serpents,
Rod of Asclepius, Medical Caduceus

The journey of this writing is about discovering *root causes of the crisis in our current medical system*, to better understand from where our dependence on these institutions really stems. Emotional thinking very rarely involves logical decision-making. This is why we had to start by appreciating the historical context in which healers arose in various societies throughout history. As doctors and physicians became more systematized, as medicine became more regulated, we can now more clearly see how modern society ended up as it is today.

However, we are not yet done combing through ancient history. There is one more civilization that changed everything as we know it, and one man who spearheaded it all, Hippocrates of Kos. The world of old was fast changing as ancient civilizations began to share written words, travel routes opened up, and religions and customs spread. However, these global changes were minor compared with the seismic rifts taking place in fifth-century BC Greece. The first forms of democracy, economic prosperity, literature, drama, and impressive architecture were all erupting in Greece during this time. Revolutions of consciousness were taking place and philosophical ideologies were being challenged.

Most people have heard of both Plato and his student Aristotle, two of the most eminent philosophers in history. Although they had a teacher-student relationship, as Aristotle aged, his thinking began to diverge from the conventional ideas of Plato and his contemporaries, who were more abstract and utopian in their philosophy. Aristotle emphasized empirical research, common sense, and practicality. Their differences can be best illustrated by the iconic *School of Athens* painting, created by Italian Renaissance painter Raphael. In this beautiful piece, we can see Plato and Aristotle walking together in conversation surrounded by philosophers, scientists, and artists of earlier and later ages. Plato, holding a copy of his dialogue *Timeo* (*Timaeus*), points upward to the heavens, while Aristotle, holding his *Etica* (*Ethics*), points outward to the world.

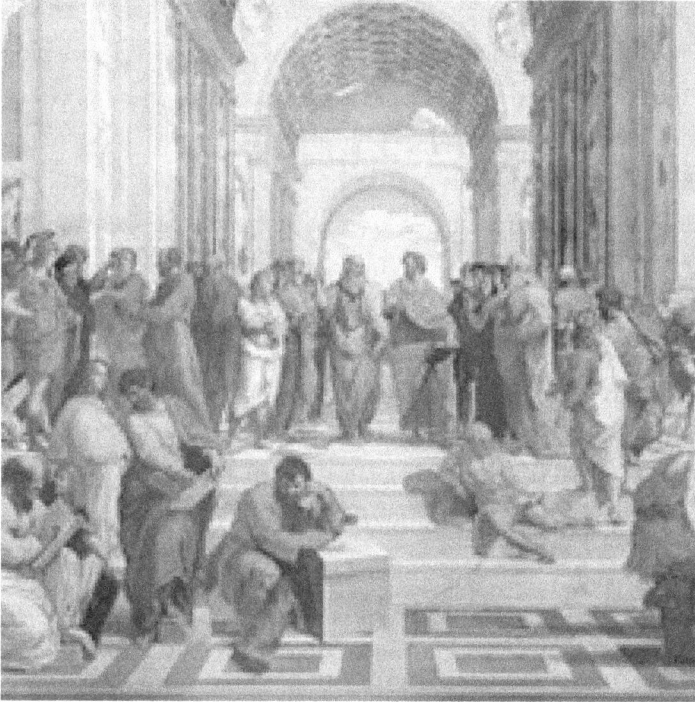

The School of Athens by Raphael 1509-1511.

Aristotle, whose father was a doctor, challenged the transcendental ideas put forth by Plato and called for the systematic observation of nature. The idea that "reality must be explained through natural causes" changed the course of science. Take Aristotle's viewpoint on health and illness, for example. Before this time, the explanations for illness and disease were supernatural and metaphysical, involving gods, spirits, or energies. As philosopher Bob Dylan wrote, "The times they are a-changin'."

This was the environment the Father of Medicine was born into, about two hundred miles south of Athens on the island of Kos. The precise details of the personal life of Hippocrates (460–370 BC), as with any iconic figure who lived thousands of years ago, are not well known. Based on numerous overlapping accounts, we do know that Hippocrates was likely born into a family of physicians and studied his craft at the Asklepion, a particular kind of healing temple found throughout Greece dedicated to the Greek god of healing, Asclepios. Despite that he was born before Aristotle, Hippocrates still subscribed to the ideology of natural causes, rejecting superstition vehemently.

This viewpoint ushered in a new era of health and medicine that would stand the test of time and directly influence history's most eminent doctors and scientists. The majority of these revolutionary concepts can be found in the *Hippocratic Corpus*, composed of sixty written texts on a variety of health topics, including systematic approaches to diagnosis, observations, treatments, stages of illness, infectious diseases, classifications of injury, fertility, hygiene, dentistry, and even neurological conditions such as epilepsy. Epilepsy is often linked with Hippocrates because his viewpoint on it perfectly highlights his disdain for the outdated philosophies of his time. In one of the books attributed to Hippocrates, *On the Sacred Disease*, he had this to say about epilepsy: "It appears to me to be nowise more divine nor more sacred than other diseases but has a natural cause like other affections. Men regard its nature and cause as divine from ignorance and wonder because it is not at all like other diseases. And this notion of its divinity is kept up by their inability to comprehend it. … Those who first referred this disease to the gods appear to me to have been just such persons as the conjurers and charlatans. … Such persons, then, using divinity as a pretext and screen of their own inability to afford any assistance, have given out that the disease is sacred."[31]

---

[31]   J. Queijo, *Breakthrough!: How the 10 Greatest Discoveries in Medicine Saved Millions and Changed Our View of the World* (FT Press Science, 2010).

Think about how significant this understanding of neurology was. Up until then, little was known about the brain and how it affects our health. Egyptians removed the brain from their revered leaders during the embalming process and threw it away! To the Egyptians, the source of all feeling, emotion, and power was the heart. Hippocratic ideology argued, "Men ought to know that the source of our pleasures, merriment, laughter, and amusements, as well as our grief, pains, anxiety, and tears, is none other than the brain."[32]

The modern consensus around the *Hippocratic Corpus* is that not all of it was written by Hippocrates. This would explain why the topics are so wide-ranging, the opinions somewhat contradictory, and the writing styles unique from topic to topic. Some experts even think that different parts of the *Hippocratic Corpus* were written hundreds of years after the death of Hippocrates, which only speaks to the legacy of Hippocrates himself. It is impossible to identify all of the writings and actions that are directly from the man Hippocrates instead of all of the students and physicians he inspired, but one thing is undeniable: Hippocrates left behind a lasting legacy in medicine that changed everything.

In this new Hippocratic era of medicine and healing, for the first time in human history, physicians had a unified code of conduct. How they should behave—the importance of ethics and personal philosophy—was now a systematic requirement for all practicing physicians and students of medicine. *On The Physician*, one of the many texts in the *Hippocratic Corpus*, goes into extensive detail about how ideal physicians should conduct

---

[32]   J. Queijo, *Breakthrough!: How the 10 Greatest Discoveries in Medicine Saved Millions and Changed Our View of the World* (FT Press Science, 2010).

themselves. The ideal doctor should be an outstanding citizen, beyond reproach or corruption, honest and moral. Their office should be clean and inviting; instruments should be laid out methodically and in a tidy manner. Hippocrates even paved the way for modern health records; he advised that all physicians should keep clean and organized notes on patients and that all new treating physicians must read through past notes to properly understand the patient's history. Many of these requirements can be found in the Hippocratic Oath. The original text, as stated in the National Library of Medicine, is as follows.

"I swear by Apollo the physician, and Asclepius, and Hygieia and Panacea and all the gods and goddesses as my witnesses, that, according to my ability and judgment, I will keep this Oath and this contract:

"To hold him who taught me this art equally dear to me as my parents … I will impart a knowledge of the art to my own sons, and those of my teachers, and to students bound by this contract and having sworn this Oath to the law of medicine, but to no others.

"I will use those dietary regimens which will benefit my patients according to my greatest ability and judgment, and I will do no harm or injustice to them.

"I will not give a lethal drug to anyone if I am asked … I will not use the knife, even upon those suffering from stones, but I will leave this to those who are trained in this craft … Into whatever homes I go, I will enter them for the benefit of the sick, avoiding any voluntary act of impropriety or corruption, including the seduction of women or men, whether they are free men or slaves.

"Whatever I see or hear in the lives of my patients, whether in connection with my professional practice or not ... I will keep secret, as considering all such things to be private.

"So long as I maintain this Oath faithfully and without corruption, may it be granted to me to partake of life fully and the practice of my art, gaining the respect of all men for all time. However, should I transgress this Oath and violate it, may the opposite be my fate."

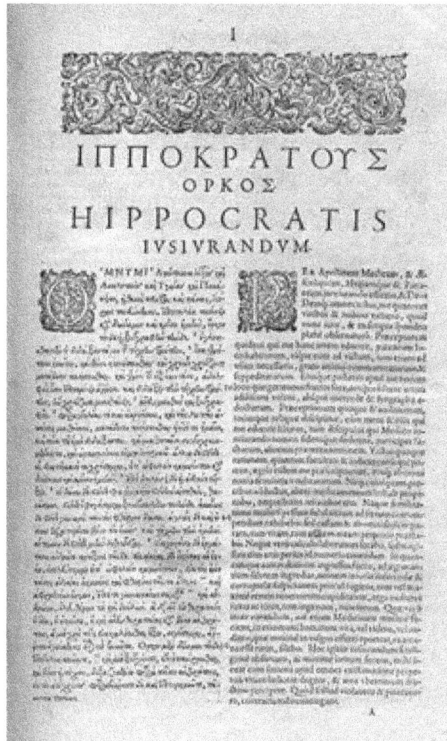

The Hippocratic Oath in Greek and Latin published in Frankfurt in 1595 in Apud Andreae Wecheli heredes.

It is one of the most influential pieces of writing on the modern world of medicine. It was rediscovered around the early 1500s in Germany, and, with minor changes to reflect a more

Christian ideology, the oath became widespread throughout Europe. Around the 1700s, the Hippocratic Oath was translated into English. After that, the spread of Hippocratic core philosophies took place all throughout Western medicine. In 1948, it was adopted by the World Medical Association and finally revised for more modern times in 1964 by Louis Lasagna, dean of the Tufts University School of Medicine. This final adaptation still holds true to the spirit of Hippocrates, promising to never overtreat and to strive for prevention. Although many of the original phrases are no longer recited, modern variations are still used by doctors and students around the world today.

By changing the way medicine was taught and practiced, Hippocrates forever changed the way the world thought about doctors. Before his work and the rise of medical schools, physicians did not hold the highest status in their communities. As healers started to diverge from having spiritual authority, their status was no longer revered. Having the ability to treat injuries and prescribe dietary regimens was seen as more of a manual labor job. Before the systematic changes by Hippocrates, there was no standard of medical care. In one town, the local healer might only have been skilled in setting fractures and closing wounds. In another town, the healer might have been versed only in topical ointments and herbal remedies. Hippocrates and his followers changed that. They brought uniformity and a standard to the world. And the world noticed. The status of physicians was substantially elevated after Hippocrates. Local governments started to allocate public funds to ensure doctors were paid for their essential work. Medical schools were built all over the place. Famous philosophers wrote about Hippocrates and his views. Physicians now had a system to follow. Hippocrates may not have had the technology available to discover cells and bacteria, like Anton van Leeuwenhoek in 1670, or the ability to process and manufacture insulin, but the systems and processes he helped instill into medicine were used to bring forth some of humankind's greatest accomplishments. Why else do we still encourage medical students to recite the Hippocratic Oath, or to keep organized medical charts, or to honor doctor-patient confidentiality?

The Hippocratic approach to medicine is clearly effective and used all over the world. But we cannot forget his approach to healing. He often chose conservative, minimalist approaches. He saw health and illness through the lens of *nature* and *balance*, defining health as "a state of dynamic equilibrium between the internal and the external environment." Illness results when this balance is upset, and thus the important thing for maintaining health is to practice a way of life that allows for minimum disturbances to occur in the body.[33]

And it seems like we could just say "the rest was history," except...medicine and health care—*somewhere* along the journey—seem to have lost their way. Unfortunately, this *simple* and *noninvasive* approach to health is no longer practiced. Health care today may operate using some of the original Hippocratic essences, but the state of our collective health is in critical condition.

And now, to honor the spirit of Sakichi Toyoda's *root cause* analysis, we must continue to ask ourselves, "Where does our clear and obvious dependence on medicine come from?" The answers to this question may not be found by analyzing the healing practices of a few thousand years ago, but doing so helps provide us with emotional context. It is now clear that medicine, in many ways, is just as old and revered as religion

---

[33]   Y. Tountas, "The Origins of Health Promotion," *Health Promotion International* 24, no. 2 (2009): 185–192.

is. We are talking about deep-seated institutions in our society. Every ambulance that speeds past you bears the same symbol that was present in ancient Egypt. Clearly, medicine offers services that are substantially different from those your local religious leaders do. However, tradition is strong in our country, for better or for worse.

From Hippocrates to Rene Laennec, Elizabeth Blackwell to Jonas Salk, medicine and healing have had a rich history. But our question remains unanswered: What happened in our country to cause such a dependence on traditional health care on a scale we have never seen before?

CHAPTER 2

FRONTIER HEALING

"I am afraid that our eyes are bigger than our stomachs,
and that we have more curiosity than understanding. We
grasp at everything but catch nothing except wind."
        —Michel de Montaigne

Egyptian priests, medicine men and women, Hippocrates and his followers—all serve as important examples of how powerful health care is as an *institution*, as well as how intertwined religion and healing have been. However, combing through records and accounts of health care providers from thousands of years ago doesn't quite help us explain the past one hundred years of policy, legislation, and social movements that have led us to a society entirely dependent on medicine.

This question emerges: What is the root cause of the current state of our health care, the fact that 66 percent of Americans are on prescription medication, and the awfully high physician and nurse burnout rates?[34] Did this all happen overnight, or was there a pivotal moment in our history that

---

[34]   Georgetown University Health Policy Institute, "Prescription Drugs," https://hpi.georgetown.edu/rxdrugs/.

shifted the momentum in this direction? If we could hop into a time machine and visit the late 1800s and early 1900s, we would see health care being practiced in an extremely different manner from how it is practiced today. Most people back then did not receive health care in a hospital setting. Those services were reserved for the destitute and marginalized. If you were considered middle to upper class by societal standards, you could easily afford to have the doctor pay you a home visit. Even some surgical procedures were done in home settings. Most hospitals during this time were a product of religious institutions in collaboration with local philanthropic groups. Many of these hospitals were not for profit, and physicians and nurses were either making very little or donating their services. Private at-home visits were much more lucrative.

Medically trained doctors and nurses weren't the only health care professionals working at the time. The osteopathic profession was well underway. Andrew Still (1828–1917) was one of nine children of a Methodist preacher and physician. The Still family was constantly on the move, as was common for many preachers at the time. Andrew was twenty-five when the family settled down in Kansas, and he decided to take up his father's profession and become a physician. He enjoyed traveling the frontier to tend to patients who had very little access to doctors, using the common practices of the day such as bleeding, blistering, and purging.[35] Less than ten years later, the Civil War was on Andrew's doorstep, and being passionate about protecting Kansas's status as a "free state," he promptly enlisted to serve as a hospital steward in the 9th Kansas Cav-

[35]   Museum of Osteopathic Medicine at A.T. Still University, "Museum," https://www.atsu.edu/museum-of-osteopathic-medicine/museum-at-still.

alry, a captain in the 18th Kansas Militia, and a major in the 21st Kansas Militia. Thankfully he was unharmed in defense of Kansas City and a battle against General Sterling Price. Whether you're a farm boy from southwestern Tennessee, a father of six in Pennsylvania, or even a family physician in Kansas City like Andrew, war leaves its marks on everyone. "War is hell," said Union General William Tecumseh Sherman. After seeing the atrocities in the Civil War, and losing his first wife to childbirth, two children to meningitis, and another child to pneumonia, Andrew Still began to question what he had learned about medicine and its abilities.

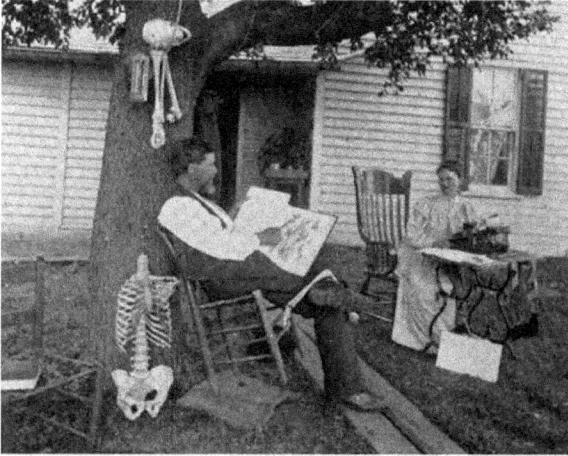

Dr. A.T. Still and his assistant, Mrs. Annie
Morris outside her residence.

Still was a man of religion and education, constantly exposing himself to the new and emerging theories of the times. In his rejection of traditional medicine, he sought out alternatives to crude surgeries and ineffective medications. It is unclear exactly which alternative methods he gravitated toward or stayed away from, but we do know that at this point in time there was growing interest in magnetic healing, bonesetting,

Grahamism, hydropathy, homeopathy, and eclecticism. It is also known that Still had an in-depth understanding of the structural relationships between bones, fascia, muscles, and ligaments. Growing up on a farm and hunting gave him many opportunities to study anatomy and the role structure plays in function. He knew that deviations in structure could adversely affect the function of a living organism and that correction of these deviations was paramount. He theorized that freeing up these deviations could drastically improve circulation and blood flow.

Not surprisingly, Andrew Still was met with fierce opposition from friends and family. They could not understand why he would be renouncing his family's legacy. Medical institutions also began to reject his presence on campus and canceled many of his speaking engagements. He bounced around from city to city in an effort to find a more accepting environment for his new form of manipulative medicine. In March of 1875, he landed in Kirksville, Missouri, advertising himself as a "magnetic healer" and "lightning bonesetter." It wasn't until 1885 that he coined the term *osteopathy*, and by then he had built quite a reputation and following.

Andrew Still founded the American School of Osteopathy (ASO) in Kirksville in 1892. By the time of his death in 1917, there were more than 3,000 osteopathic medical doctors. Three years after the death of their beloved founder, the A.T. Still Research Institute of Pasadena put forth a code of osteopathic principles that was widely adopted by practicing physicians in the profession.

1. The body is a unit (of mind, body, and spirit).
2. The body is in fact capable of self-healing, regulating, and maintenance.
3. Structure and function are reciprocally interrelated.

4. Rational treatment is based on an understanding of these principles: body unity, self-regulation, and the interrelationship of structure and function.[36]

It was the innovative introduction of anatomical manipulation and principles that set osteopathic physicians apart from conventional medical doctors. Before shifting societal and political tides, thousands of patients warmly embraced this emerging profession.

At a glance, osteopathic medicine looks similar to another well-known healing profession, chiropractic, which was founded in Davenport, Iowa, ten years *after* osteopathy, by Daniel David Palmer. Palmer, referred to as D. D., was exposed to philosophies nearly identical to those that had influenced Andrew Still. D. D. also participated in magnetic healing and was familiar with bonesetting. Born in 1845 in Ontario, Canada, D. D. moved to the United States when he was twenty-five years old, ending up in Burlington and Davenport, Iowa, where he built up his eclectic healing practice—a combination of spiritualism, magnetic healing, and various hands-on approaches.

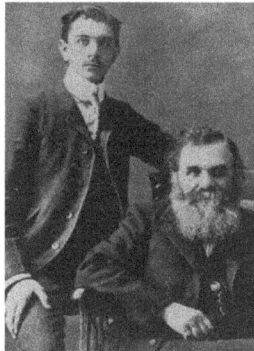

Daniel David Plamer (D.D.)
and son Bartlett Joshua Palmer (B.J.)

---

[36] Norman Gevitz, "The Future of Osteopathic Principles," *J Am Osteopath Assoc* 106, no. 3 (2006): 121–129.

D. D.'s fixation was on the novel concept of *inflammation* and how it seemed to be the culprit behind all diseases in the body. In 1895 and early 1896, he was declaring inflammation to be formed by displaced anatomy.[37] Now, through the use of his hands and based on nine years of clinical experience, he was putting his theories to the test. Another tenant in the Ryan building where D. D. practiced was a man named Harvey Lillard, the owner of the building's janitorial business. Whether Lillard approached Palmer or the other way around is unclear, but the two met and began to discuss Lillard's health. Lillard had been nearly deaf for many years after a back injury, which he recounted as being accompanied by a "cracking" sensation. After examining Lillard's spine, D. D. identified a rather large lump of inflamed tissue, and his theories around health centering on healthy anatomy led him to take specific and guided action. On September 18, 1895, D. D. Palmer gave the first recorded chiropractic adjustment to Harvey Lillard. Two years later, Lillard wrote a testimonial published in a local paper titled "The Chiropractic."

"I was deaf for 17 years and I expected to always remain so, for I had doctored a great deal without any benefit. I had long ago made up my mind to not take any more ear treatments, for it did me no good. Last January Dr. Palmer told me that my deafness came from an injury in my spine. This was new to me; but it is a fact that my back was injured at the time I went deaf. Dr. Palmer treated me on the spine; in two treatments I could hear quite well. That was eight months ago. My hearing remains good."

---

[37] Joseph C. Keating, Carl S. Cleveland, and Michael Menke, *Chiropractic History: A Primer* (Association for the History of Chiropractic, 2004).

my mother-in-law and brother-in-law of
heart disease. Our family have reasons for thinking well of your cures.
        MRS. NELLIE RICHARDSON,
September 10, 1896.   Lake City, Iowa.

DEAF SEVENTEEN YEARS.

I was deaf 17 years and I expected
to always remain so, for I had doctored
a great deal without any benefit. I
had long ago made up my mind to not
take any more ear treatments, for it
did me no good.
    Last January Dr. Palmer told me
that my deafness came from an injury
in my spine. This was new to me;
but it is a fact that my back was injured at the time I went deaf. Dr.
Palmer treated me on the spine; in
two treatments I could hear quite well.
That was eight months ago. My hearing remains good.
                HARVEY LILLARD,
320 W. Eleventh St., Davenport, Iowa.

Harvey Lillard's healing testimony of his
first chiropractic adjustment.

D. D. Palmer, with the help of his friend and patient Rev.
Samuel Weed, had coined the name of *chiropractic*, meaning
"done by hand," for his new practice. Palmer opened a teaching
clinic in the building he was working out of. The year 1896 saw
the first students coming out of Palmer's School of Chiropractic, including his son, Bartlett Joshua (B. J.) Palmer. Several
of the graduates were also allopathic and osteopathic doctors.

Chiropractic and osteopathy shared many features in their
early days. In addition to methods of intervening and a holistic approach, they both had political and legal battles on
the way to becoming legitimate healing professions. Always
under harassment and persecution by medical organizations,

practitioners were commonly summoned to appear in courts to testify on their own behalf. This is one reason why D. D. left his position at the Palmer School of Chiropractic in 1902, leaving its leadership to his son B. J., and he made his way to Santa Barbara, California, to teach.

D. D. further developed his theories on healing in 1903, abandoning his first theory—that inflammation is a consequence of displaced anatomy: arteries, veins, nerves, muscles, bones, ligaments, joints, or any anatomic structure that is out of its normal position. He had now reduced his anatomical focus to joints only, especially those in the spine. Palmer believed that when these joints misaligned, or to use his word, *subluxated*, they could irritate the nerve roots as they exited the vertebral foramina (small openings). Palmer thought that pressure on these nerves would cause increased neural impulses to be sent to the organs they fed into, thus causing inflammation.[38] The Palmers would continue to tweak and revise their theories for the next several years, all the while promoting subluxation as their primary focus. It is important to note that this transition from theory number one to theory number two, focusing on the nervous system and the spine, was instrumental in clearly distinguishing chiropractic from the all-too-similar osteopathy and teachings of Andrew Still.

---

[38] Joseph C. Keating, Carl S. Cleveland, and Michael Menke, *Chiropractic History: A Primer* (Association for the History of Chiropractic, 2004).

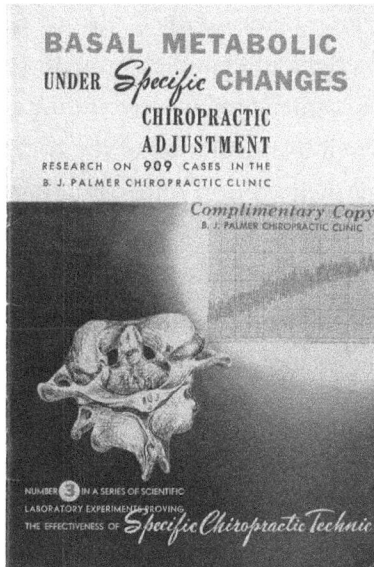

Examples of research being conducted through
the B.J. Palmer Chiropractic Clinic

One guiding principle of chiropractic that has endured
over a hundred years is the concept of *innate intelligence*. D. D.
postulated that innate intelligence is an inborn mechanism that
directs all the functions of the body and uses the nervous system to exert its influence. This concept undoubtedly distances
chiropractic from any allopathic health care profession, further
bolstering chiropractic ownership of *vitalism*, the doctrine that
living organisms are sustained by a nonphysical vital force.

Under the leadership of B. J., the Palmer School of Chiropractic continued to flourish. More schools around the country
began to teach the science, philosophy, and art of chiropractic,
and the profession was growing. B. J., affectionately referred to
as the "developer of chiropractic," was quick to implement new
and emerging science and technology to improve the discipline
of chiropractic whenever possible. In 1910, Palmer, with great
enthusiasm, introduced X-ray technology to the profession. In

the Palmer Research Institute, there already lay thousands of osteological collections and samples, primarily of spines, which aided in the advancement and understanding of spinal biomechanics. With the implementation of the X-ray, chiropractors were able to take their clinical understanding of subluxation to the next level. In 1924, B. J. introduced the *neurocalometer*, a two-pronged spinal heat-sensing instrument to more accurately detect subluxation. Although many chiropractors initially protested its use, this was the beginning of a long line of technological advancements.

Also prominent in the health care scene was the profession of naturopathy. Although its primary belief, that nature holds a healing power (*vis medicatrix naturae*), can be traced all the way back to Hippocrates, the formal organization and standard practices of naturopathy are much more modern, dating back to Germany in the 1800s. At a time when many alternative forms of healing were emerging—such as hydrotherapy, natural cure movement, and homeopathy—Benedict Lust, considered to be the father of American naturopathy, sought out the help of a well-known Catholic priest. When Lust contracted tuberculosis in 1892, he traveled back to Germany, his country of birth, to receive healing from the renowned priest Father Sebastian Kneipp. Father Kneipp used primarily hydrotherapy to restore Lust to health. Lust, who claimed to have been cured by these sessions, returned to the United States a fierce advocate for all of Father Kneipp's healing modalities. In 1901, Lust founded the American School of Naturopathy and instituted the Naturopathic Societies.[39]

---

[39]   P. Snider and J. Zeff, "Unifying Principles of Naturopathic Medicine: Origins and Definitions," *Integrative Medicine (Encinitas)* 18, no. 4 (2019): 36–39.

Lust, being a passionate proponent of anything natural, took up studies in osteopathy and chiropractic, and in 1905 he even started his own chiropractic school. As the profession of naturopathy blossomed, it quickly spread across the country. After only a few years, naturopathic physicians could obtain licensure to practice in twenty-five states. State-sanctioned licensure was critical to these young health care fields. Licensure in many ways helped solidify the status of these physicians as credible, professional, and genuine health care providers.

At this time, when health care in the country was like the Wild West, it was hard to know whether you were soliciting the services of a rural country medical doctor, a qualified naturopathic doctor, an osteopath, or an individual who was knowingly selling deceptive cures for various ailments. We know the last group of individuals as "snake oil salesmen," slick operators who could be found in every town touting their latest cure for any current ailment, and they were master marketers! At the height of the manufacturing and distribution of these "cures," ads for patent medicines accounted for roughly half of newspapers' entire advertising income. The ingredients for these patent medicines were kept secret and sold under trademarked names such as Lydia E. Pinkham's Vegetable Compound, Hamlin's Wizard Oil, Kickapoo Indian Sagwa, and Warner's Safe Diabetes Cure.[40] The main ingredient in these tonics, salves, and bitters was water, with varying amounts of alcohol or opium. The claims the salesmen made were typically false and even dangerous. For instance, Lydia E. Pinkham's Vegetable Compound claimed "to cure entirely the worst form of female complaints, all ovarian troubles, Inflammation and Ulceration, Falling and

---

[40]   Julie Donohue, "A History of Drug Advertising: The Evolving Roles of Consumers and Consumer Protection," *The Milbank Quarterly* 84, no. 4 (2006): 659–699.

Displacements."[41] Health care in America during the late 1800s and early 1900s was indeed a wild scenario, but for better or for worse, a new sheriff was rolling into town.

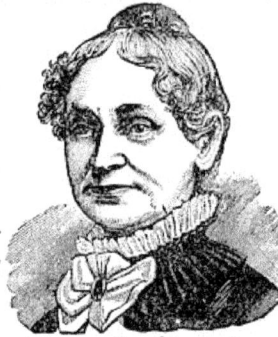

Advertisement for Lydia E. Pinkham's Vegetable Compound 1882. One of the many kinds of "patent medicines" of the day.

---

[41]   Julie Donohue, "A History of Drug Advertising: The Evolving Roles of Consumers and Consumer Protection," *The Milbank Quarterly* 84, no. 4 (2006): 659–699.

CHAPTER 3

A MEDICAL TRANSFORMATION

"We are all born brave, trusting, and greedy, and most of us remain greedy."

—Mignon McLaughlin

THE TECHNOLOGICAL REVOLUTION in America between 1890 and 1903 was seismic. The introduction of the radio brought millions of Americans together, and by 1920, over 100 million radios were in use. In 1893, Frank and Charles Duryea of Springfield, Massachusetts, designed the first successful American gasoline automobile, and by 1910, around 500,000 motor vehicles were being driven all over the country. On December 17, 1903, two brothers by the name of Wright made four brief flights on their gasoline-powered aircraft, thus inventing the first successful airplane. This technological revolution ignited a social and cultural revolution in America that would soon spread to every facet of society. Americans now had an insatiable taste for innovation. They wanted better, faster, more efficient *everything*. Clearly, cutting-edge thinking has the ability to drastically improve our well-being. We were now able to drive, fly, and connect with the world for the first time in human history! It was also time to apply these principles to health care in America.

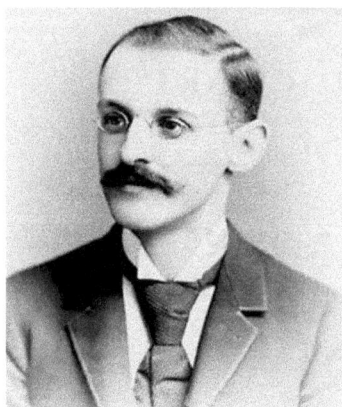

Photograph of Abraham Flexner

Thus, the Hopkins Circle was formed. William Welch, the founding dean at Johns Hopkins University, and William Osler, the first chief of medicine at Hopkins, sat on this council. Also in its membership was Baptist minister and trusted adviser to John D. Rockefeller Frederick Gates, whose role was to serve as the go-between for the Hopkins Circle and Rockefeller, convincing him to provide the financial resources to ensure the group's success. Soon the group enlisted the help of one final member, Abraham Flexner, a former high school teacher and expert on public education. After obtaining a two-year degree from Johns Hopkins University, he quickly gained a large public following and admiration for his unique approach to education, which introduced student-led problem-solving rather than the outdated model of simple memorization. Flexner eventually made his way to England, France, and Germany, where he took particular notice of differing philosophies on education and obtained the additional needed perspective to write his book *The American College.* This book, largely a critique of modern American education that offered solutions, caught the attention of Henry Pritchett, head of the Carnegie Foundation.[42]

Remember, this happened in the midst of the technological revolution. The major corporations and industries throughout the country were in a race to create and distribute the next innovative masterpiece, and health care was ripe for the taking. Perhaps this is one reason the Carnegie Foundation and the Rockefeller family had taken quite the sudden interest in medicine. And so the invitation was extended to Abraham Flexner to survey the quality of medical schools throughout America and Canada. In response, Flexner created a report in which he outlined his criticisms and provided solutions he deemed necessary to improve the country's quality of medical doctors.

But why Abraham Flexner? Isn't it odd that the country's most influential philanthropists and doctors were placing this task in the hands of someone who was *not* a doctor, who had never even set foot in a medical school? Perhaps the Hopkins Circle diagnosed the problem of medical education as an *educational* problem and not a medical problem. More probably, they knew that these soon-to-be-published critiques would likely be met with pushback and resentment, and maybe the fact that Abraham Flexner was not a physician would mitigate the backlash. Whatever their reasons, Flexner was enlisted to tour the country, analyze as many teaching programs as he could, and essentially stamp out any and all "substandard" medical schools (and practices) that were contributing to the increasingly poor quality of American physicians. Fortunately

---

[42]   Thomas P. Duffy, "The Flexner Report—100 Years Later," *The Yale Journal of Biology and Medicine* 84, no. 3 (2011): 269–276.

for Flexner, the Carnegie Foundation, and the Rockefeller family, he was wildly successful in these endeavors, and he even went back to Germany a second time before publishing his official report. Unfortunately for the rest of the United States, the 1910 publication of *Medical Education in the United States and Canada* initiated the monumental decline of almost all other forms of health care in this country. No one can debate the benefits to humankind that modern medicine and research have provided, but what were the unintended, unfortunate consequences of this report for millions of Americans?

Let's start with the Flexner report's *intended* consequences. The faults of American medical education were obvious: no standards, poor regulatory boards, poor oversight, and very little laboratory and research experience. Flexner knew where he wanted to start with his reform. By using the German model as his prototype, his main goal was to make *science* the primary focus. Medical students were to devote far more time to the scientific investigation of diseases, and as in Germany, physicians and students alike were to be made responsible for the contribution of new information and progress in medical science. How did Flexner suggest America make the switch to this new ideal physician?

Full-time teaching. Up until then, medical-school professors both taught and actively saw patients. The bulk of a medical-school teacher's salary came from treating patients. Flexner, the educator that he was, saw major room for improving the quality of education by freeing professors from their patient-care responsibilities to devote themselves to full-time instructing. An incredible influx of cash flowed into the medical schools (primarily via the Carnegie Foundation and Rockefeller family) to ensure that professors could receive the necessary income to focus solely on academics. A. McGehee Harvey, chairman of the Department of Medicine at Johns Hopkins, went on record saying he believed that this change in policy had made the single most profound effect on medical education and medical practice.[43]

However, there were staunch opponents to this policy. Ironically enough, William Osler and his mentee Harvey Cushing were incredibly vocal in their misgivings about this new approach. Osler believed that it would cause the focus of medical physicians to become too narrow and compartmentalized. He feared what would happen to the quality of care if teaching professors became disconnected from their own patients' lives. Educating students on the welfare of patients should be the top priority, rather than the advancement of knowledge for the sake of knowledge. Osler and Cushing were not alone in their reservations; however, they were hardly heard in the face of the enticing prospect of the great amounts of money poised to flow into medical schools.

Medicine now had a new emotional appeal. Science was to be the gold standard. The goal of medical academia would be to advance clinical understanding and pave new ground. On paper, this sounds beautiful. And this new guiding compass did lead to many lifesaving achievements. Too many to list. However, these were all the *intended* consequences. Abraham Flexner had created a three-tiered grading system for medical schools. The first group he deemed as "suitable and up to standard." The second tier he deemed "salvageable with some financial donations and restructuring." The third group he deemed "poor quality," and he recommended that they

---

[43]   Thomas P. Duffy, "The Flexner Report—100 Years Later," *The Yale Journal of Biology and Medicine* 84, no. 3 (2011): 269–276.

be closed. After his report was published, over one-third of medical schools were indeed closed in America. But this was the least damaging consequence of the Carnegie-Rockefeller sponsored report.

If we wish to truly understand *when* our demand for "modern medicine" really began, where the *root cause* of today's problem with health care is, it's in the years following 1910. This is when the United States saw a tremendous decline in health care diversity. For the first time in the history of the world, a monopoly on healing existed. The few remaining medical-teaching institutions in the country, backed by large corporations and wealthy sponsors, had the ability to create a homogenized way of thinking about health. They could set the standards for what passed, and did not pass, as health care. Organizations such as the American Medical Association (AMA) were now the primary regulatory and oversight entities, granting medical licenses and ensuring that standards of medical practices were upheld. The key word there is *medical* practices. Unfortunately, the aftermath of the Flexner Report was not only medicine's monopoly of health care but also the decimation of health professions such as naturopathy, osteopathy (to an extent), and most notably, the chiropractic profession.

Let's start with naturopathy. Within just the first three decades of naturopathy's arrival in the United States, the profession was able to establish a strong foothold. Naturopaths were licensed to practice in twenty-five states. Because of the philosophies on health shared by chiropractors and naturopaths, several chiropractic programs throughout the country began to offer naturopathic degrees for students who wished to practice both disciplines. But the situation went downhill just as quickly. The Flexner Report had further emboldened the AMA crackdown on everything "nonmedical" as it pertained to such things as licensing laws, scope of practice, and school accreditation. The Flexner Report placed the science of medicine above all else, stigmatizing the sciences found within osteopathy, naturopathy, and chiropractic. Less than thirty years after the country shifted its stance on health care, there were only five states in which naturopaths could obtain licensure.[44] Because of the pressure the AMA was placing on the chiropractic profession, nearly all chiropractic programs stopped offering ND degrees to students.

The newly acquired stigma on "holistic" or "alternative" healing professions made it hard for practitioners to maintain professional authority. Many naturopathic doctors regularly used homeopathic remedies and supplements. Of course, these were not new methods and practices. Cultures around the world have been using herbal and natural remedies for thousands of years, but, for the first time, negative connotations were being attached to them. Whether because of the lack of medical-standard research or the simultaneous emergence of highly effective medications (such as penicillin), the interest in pursuing natural cures and remedies was in rapid decline. In 1968, the United States government created a task force to survey health care to determine what should and should not be covered by Medicare and Medicaid. Their report included harsh criticisms of naturopathy, claiming that it was not rooted in medical science and that its scope was too large. The task force concluded by saying, "In view of the findings of the 1968

---

[44] Hans A. Baer, "The Sociopolitical Status of U.S. Naturopathy at the Dawn of the 21st Century," *Medical Anthropology Quarterly* 15 (2001): 329–346.

study, the Task Force concludes that payment for such services is not an effective use of Federal Medicaid funds."[45]

Although osteopathy fared much better in the long run than naturopathy, the young profession nevertheless had a tumultuous journey. Why? Because it was going against the grain of traditional medicine and rejecting much of allopathic medicine's philosophy. The Flexner Report significantly catapulted allopathic medicine to the high social status it has today and made great efforts in stamping out other health professions. Furthermore, allopathic medicine was coming in on the coattails of an existing group that was already actively waging war against holistic approaches to health care: the AMA.

---

[45] *Report of the Task Force on Medicaid and Related Programs* (U.S. Department of Health, Education, and Welfare, 1970).

CHAPTER 4

THE UPHILL BATTLES

"Nothing reduces the odds against you like ignoring them."
—Robert Breault

THE AMERICAN MEDICAL Association is a countrywide professional and lobbying group comprising medical students and practicing physicians. Founded in 1847 by Dr. Nathan Smith Davis, the group's main objective at that time was to bring about systems and procedures to improve the quality of care and record-keeping throughout the country. A major early achievement was a code of ethics—with a focus on legislation aimed at regulating the production of harmful, ineffective "patent medicines." Thus, the Drug Importation Act of 1848 was passed.[46]

The AMA had now realized its strength and effectiveness in numbers and gradually began to set its sights on any and all competition in the marketplace. The group may have had pure intentions originally (protection of the well-being of Americans, shielding them from harmful snake oil salesmen and the like),

---

[46]   Bob Zebroski, *A Brief History of Pharmacy: Humanity's Search for Wellness* (Routledge, 2015).

but their efforts turned into an all-out persecution of homeo-paths, naturopaths, osteopaths, and chiropractors. The collec-tive crime of these professions? Using science and techniques that fell outside of the scope and practice of *medical* science and techniques. There was more concern for the divergence from standard medical practices than for the actual well-being of patients. Consider homeopathy for example.

In 1844, thirty-one years before the emergence of oste-opathy, the American Institute of Homeopathy was founded. Homeopathic practitioners received no mercy from the AMA. Being the primary competitor to medicine at the time, any nonorthodox physicians began to be referred to by the AMA as "quacks".[47] The AMA also began to refer to its own practice of medicine (which back then was still extremely crude) as "scientific medicine," further differentiating medical doctors from so-called quacks.

From its inception, osteopathy faced much adversity in even obtaining licenses from state health boards. DOs—doc-tors of osteopathy—could be heavily persecuted for practicing their profession unless they had proper licensing and certifica-tion (which, oddly enough, was being granted only by medical professionals). Think about how bizarre that is. Members of the AMA sat on every major state board when it came to legislation and regulation of various health professions. For several years in New York, there were heated debates as to the legitimacy of osteopathic medicine and its educational requirements. The state legislature was angling to push out osteopaths altogether.

However, an unlikely hero came to the aid of DOs. In 1901, Mark Twain stood before the New York Committee on

---

[47]   Paul S. Boyer, *The Oxford Companion to United States History* (Oxford: Oxford University Press, 2004).

Public Health, proclaiming, "I don't know as I cared much about these osteopaths until I heard you were going to drive them out of the state, but since I heard that I haven't been able to sleep."[48] His statement came amid a series of debates the committee had been having on licensing rights. Several physicians in attendance aggressively retorted to Mr. Twain, which prompted his famous rebuttal, "Physicians think they are moved by regard for the best interests of the public. Isn't there a little touch of self-interest back of it all? The objection is *people are curing people without a license* and *you are afraid it will bust up business.*"

The years following the Flexner Report proved to be just as challenging for the osteopathic profession because the stigma on *alternative* health care was rising steadily. Events during World Wars I and II perfectly demonstrated the government's feelings toward osteopathic doctors. For instance, during WWI, the Selective Service Act of 1917 was passed, requiring young men between eighteen and forty-five to enlist into the armed services. Exemptions were made for a few select populations such as federal and state officials and judges, religious ministers, seminary students, and occupations deemed "essential" to the well-being of the country. Medical doctors (and medical students) fit into the "reserved occupation" category, meaning that, if medical students continued their studies, they would not be thrown into active duty. Then, if they wished, they could take the required exams to become commissioned as army physicians. This privilege was not extended to osteopathic students. The result? Thousands of students studying

---

[48]   K. P. Ober, "The Pre-Flexnerian Reports: Mark Twain's Criticism of Medicine in the United States," *Annals of Internal Medicine* 126, no. 2 (1997): 157–163.

to become osteopathic doctors were suddenly pulled from their schooling and placed in the trenches on the Western Front.

To add more insult to injury, the Medical Corps of the US War Department barred already licensed DOs from taking the exams to become commissioned in the army. Even the rare few DOs who were allowed to take the exam and passed, proving they were just as competent as their medical counterparts, were still denied commission to serve and treat the men fighting in Europe. This intentional exclusion was so egregious that in 1918, George A. Still (grandnephew of the American School of Osteopathy founder, Andrew Still) and Dr. G. W. Riley, American Osteopathic Association president, came before the US House of Representatives' Committee on Military Affairs to appeal these policies. Their objective was simple: they wanted *equal treatment* under the current laws of examination. Dr. Riley, in front of Congress, was recorded saying: "We appreciate the fact … [that] we are placing ourselves wholly in the hands of those who are avowedly and unreservedly opposed to us professionally. But … because we feel it our duty to render the best service in our power, and because we are confident that we can render a service of inestimable value to the men in the service, we unhesitatingly propose this equality of testing of our work."[49]

This appeal before Congress successfully secured the osteopaths' ability to take the examinations required for the military commission. Unfortunately, Surgeon General Gorgas and the Medical Corps had the final say on admission. Following the congressional hearing, twenty-five osteopathic doctors were allowed to take that exam. All twenty-five DOs passed with

49 Shawn A. Silver, "Thanks, But No Thanks: How Denial of Osteopathic Service in World War I and World War II Shaped the Profession," *Journal of Osteopathic Medicine* 112, no. 2 (2012): 93–97.

excellent grades and were recommended for service by their local medical boards. And all twenty-five osteopathic physicians were denied entrance, with the following explanation mailed to them: "While the law does not specifically provide that a physician, in order to enter the Medical Corps must be a Doctor of Medicine, unwritten practice does, and the Secretary of War [Newton Baker] has decided … that he will require a man coming into the Medical Corps shall have the degree of MD."[50]

Even after the First World War came to an end, anti-osteopathic sentiments continued to grow. During the 1920s, the AMA was labeling osteopaths as "cultists," and hospitals around the country began to deny staffing privileges to DOs. And then in 1923, the AMA publicly announced that it was considered dishonorable for medical doctors to consult with osteopathic doctors. Fifteen years later, the AMA began to forbid professional relationships between medical doctors and osteopaths. It's no wonder that when the Second World War broke out, osteopaths were still ineligible for commissioned service with the military Medical Corps. Thankfully, they were exempt from the draft and were able to complete their studies while thousands of medical doctors left to serve on the front lines of the war.

Consider how devastating the AMA's actions were for doctors of medicine and osteopathy, who simply wished to better the lives of their patients. Think of the people who were massively benefiting from seeing their local DO and then reading printed publications calling their doctor a cultist. This intentional effort to denigrate an entire profession was not based on science or research. The AMA, empowered by the Flexner Report, was aggressively making strides to further their

---

[50]   *The Journal of the American Osteopathic Association*, "Did the Association Fail Its Country?" 40, no. 3 (1940): 153.

medicine's monopoly on health care. The AMA was limiting and prohibiting access to any providers who did not fall under the umbrella of medicine (by their definition). And most devastating of all, they were manipulating the thinking of everyday Americans who were just trying to live healthier lives and actively participate in that effort.

CHIROPRACTIC FINED $350

Dr. D. D. Palmer Found Guilty of Practicing Without License.

Dr. D. D. Palmer, the Davenport chiropractic operator, was found guilty in the district court at Davenport of practicing medicine without a license, and was fined $350. The maximum fine is $500. Dr. Palmer says he will lay the fine out in jail, thus resigning himself to 105 days behind the bars. Though Dr. Palmers' case has been up before justice courts several times, this is the first time it has been brought in the district court.

A notice from the 1906 Rock Island Argus, announcing that D.D. Palmer was found guilty of practicing without a medical license.

There is no more flagrant illustration of the AMA's deliberate effort to eradicate competition than their crusade against the *chiropractic* profession. Before the 1910 Flexner publication, chiropractors were still facing an uphill battle, primarily in their attempt to distinguish themselves from the practice of osteopathy. To the average patient in the 1900s, it was entirely too easy to confuse a visit with a chiropractor with one to an osteopath. The difference came down entirely to intent and philosophical understanding. Remember, chiropractic was founded and developed by focusing on the nervous system and how the spine specifically can affect the nervous system via the spinal nerve roots and the spinal cord. Osteopaths, still a branch of medicine, but with a much more holistic viewpoint, mobilized many parts of the body to free up circulation. Osteopathic doctors did not limit themselves to the spine—they still included the use of medicine, and in some cases minor surgery, in their practice. These differences were of no importance to the local state medical boards, who were actively imprisoning chiropractors and accusing them of practicing medicine without a license.

Because of the high incidence of chiropractors being locked up, B. J. Palmer and several other prominent chiropractors founded the Universal Chiropractors' Association (UCA) for the sole purpose of raising money and resources to legally fight these persecutions. One of the most notable court battles took place in 1906 in Wisconsin between Palmer graduate Dr. Shegataro Morikubo and the district attorney for LaCrosse, Wisconsin. The claim? That Dr. Morikubo, a chiropractor, was practicing medicine and osteopathic medicine without a degree. Representing Dr. Morikubo was Wisconsin Senator Tom Morris.

MEDICAL ASSOCIATION
OPPOSES RECOGNITION

House of Delegates Turns Down Plan to Recognize Chiropractors and Others to Aid Them in Getting State Examination.

Shall regular practitioners as represented by the membership of the state medical association recognize magnetic healers and chiropractors even enough to aid the state association of osteopaths in securing the passage of a law which will put the non-medical practitioners all under the same board of examiners, namely, the osteopathic board? The legisla-

Dr. Wilson withdrew the objectionable part of his report but not until he had spoken his mind. Some of the doctors had said any co-ordination with the osteopaths would be undignified on the part of the state medical association. Dr. Wilson said the association had gone to seed in its dignified attitude towards the world. It had lost ground in consequence. It had opposed homeopathy, the eclectic school, and the osteopaths and had done its best to prevent recognition. But all

Headline in the Lincoln Journal Star May 12, 1914

After Morris's explanation that Dr. Morikubo was only using his hands to help his patients, the charge of "practicing medicine" was dropped. The trial then proceeded with only one accusation against the calm and humble chiropractor, "practicing osteopathy without a degree." Several osteopaths and chiropractors took the stand to patiently and clearly lay out the differences between chiropractors and osteopaths in both their theories and their hands-on practices. In addition to verbal testimony, Morris read passages from chiropractic textbooks, which also supported their defense. After a long, grueling twenty-three minutes, Dr. Morikubo was acquitted. This was the first of many wins for the chiropractic profession. Senator Morris dedicated the rest of his life to the UCA, sitting as their top legal counsel. Just as with the inception of the osteopathic profession and its struggle, obtaining "separate and distinct" licensing laws and boards of chiropractic examiners was the only way to ensure the end of these legal harassments from state medical boards.

Between 1913 (when the first state—Kansas—passed a chiropractic statute) and 1974 (when the last state—Louisiana—passed its statute), hundreds of arrests had taken place. Chiropractors had stumbled upon an interesting realization: If a chiropractor was arrested with the accusation of "practicing medicine without a license," there were two options. Pay a fine to the state or serve jail time. Often the paid fines would end up in the hands of the local state medical boards and the AMA. Chiropractors who went to jail were able to deny their medical tyrants of any financial gains. For example, in one single year—1932—California saw 450 jail sentences served by chiropractors, many of whom served multiple sentences. Chiropractors knew that there was a social movement happening throughout the country. Every time a doctor of chiropractic was removed from his or her town and put behind bars, it was the patients who truly suffered. And chiropractors knew they were winning the public's support. Why else would their patients follow them to jail and receive care?

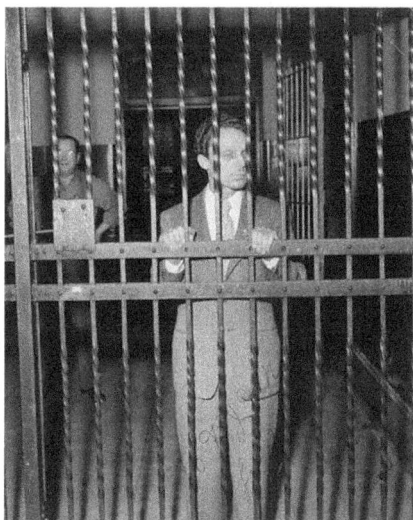

Dr. Herbert Ross Reaver was jailed 12 times—each for
the charge of "practicing medicine without a license."

The AMA had superior organizing, greater numbers,
greater political influence, and a significant war chest. Fully
employed to delay the spread of the chiropractic profession.
Despite the great disadvantages they faced, chiropractors were
licensed in forty states by 1935, and by 1961, in forty-six. Unfortunately, their struggle was just beginning. After years of
rapid growth and securing their own licensure, the chiropractic
profession was presenting itself to be more of a problem for the
AMA to handle than previously expected. In 1963, the AMA
intensified its strategies, forming the Committee on Quackery.
The methods of attack were wide-ranging, but the objective for
forming this committee was simple: "First the containment of
chiropractic and, ultimately, the elimination of chiropractic."[51]

---

[51]   Claire D. Johnson and Bart N. Green, "Looking Back at the Lawsuit
That Transformed the Chiropractic Profession Part 4: Committee on
Quackery," *Journal of Chiropractic Education* 35, no. S1 (2021): 55–73.

M E M O R A N D U M

```
TO:        Board of Trustees

FROM:      Committee on Quackery:  Joseph A. Sabatier, Jr., M.D., Chairman
                                   H. Thomas Ballantine, M.D.
                                   Clarence H. Denser, Jr., M.D.
                                   Henry I. Fineberg, M.D.
                                   David B. Stevens, M.D.
                                   H. Doyl Taylor, Secretary

DATE:      January 4, 1971
```

Since the AMA Board of Trustees' decision, at its meeting on November 2-3, 1963, to establish a Committee on Quackery, your Committee has considered its prime mission to be, first, the containment of chiropractic and, ultimately, the elimination of chiropractic.

A memo from the American Medical Association's Committee on Quackery revealed that one of its main goals was "to contain and ultimately eliminate chiropractic."

According to court documents and records from the AMA, the anti-chiropractic campaign sought to achieve several objectives: Suppress research favorable to chiropractic, undermine chiropractic colleges and postgraduate education programs, use new ethical rulings to prevent cooperation between MDs and chiropractors in education, research, and practice, subvert a 1967 United States government inquiry into the merits of chiropractic, and base an extensive misinformation campaign against chiropractic on the calculated portrayal of chiropractors as 'unscientific,' 'cultist,' and having a philosophy incompatible with western scientific medicine. Yes, chiropractors were now able to receive independent licensure in almost all fifty states and were no longer subjected to harassment from state medical boards for practicing medicine without a license. Sadly, however, this was not the only arena in which chiropractors were vulnerable. Through its broad-spectrum attack on chiropractic, the AMA began to target education. Preventing accreditation of chiropractic schools, as it had in New York, was one effective measure it pursued. And just as it had done with the naturopaths, it ensured that chiropractors would not receive any coverage through the Medicare program introduced by Congress in the 1960s.

While chiropractic associations were occupied with these new challenges, a variety of religious and alternative health groups throughout the country were just as frustrated with the AMA and decided to act. Dubbing their action Operation Sore Throat, several individuals broke into the AMA's headquarters in Chicago and photocopied confidential documents outlining unethical activities. Several of these documents were put together in a 1972 book titled *In the Public Interest*, authored by William Trever. Copies of this book were sent all around the country, making headlines in several media outlets, such as *The New York Times*. After the damning evidence was released, even more recovered documents from the AMA were leaked, landing in the hands of government officials, news reporters, and, you guessed it, chiropractic associations.

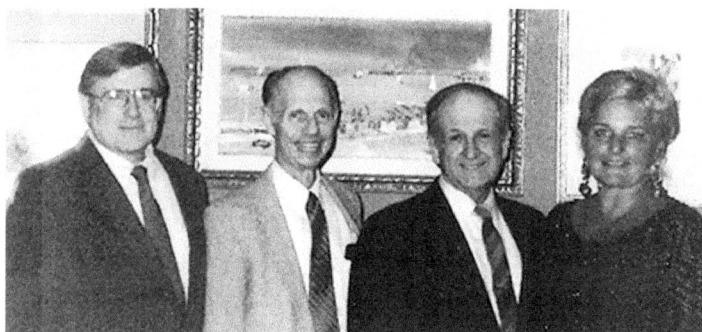

From left to right, the four chiropractors who served as plaintiffs: Michael Pedigo, James Bryden, Chester Wilk, and Patricia Arthur.

Three years after this revelation, and continued denial by the AMA, *The New York Times* published an article on October 29, 1975, stating, "The staff of the House Oversight and Investigation subcommittee has concluded that the campaign of the American Medical Association to eliminate chiropractic service in the United States may violate the antitrust laws." All these documents were compiled by the subcommittee and sent to the Federal Trade Commission (FTC) for review. This came as a relief to the chiropractic profession. Litigation was extremely expensive, requiring careful strategy as well as cohesion across the profession, which, at the time, chiropractors did not possess. Had the FTC decided to take this issue on, the chiropractors would have been spared. However, despite overwhelming evidence, the FTC decided not to take any action, forcing the chiropractic profession to step in.

Chicago-based chiropractor Chester A. Wilk and co-plaintiffs filed their suit on October 12, 1976, in the Northern District of Illinois, Eastern Division. Unbeknownst to these chiropractors, they were about to take on a fourteen-year struggle against one of the world's oldest and most powerful institutions, organized medicine. The defendants? The American Hospital Association, the American College of Surgeons, the American College of Physicians, the Joint Commission on Accreditation of Hospitals, the American College of Radiology, the American Academy of Orthopedic Surgeons, the Illinois State Medical Society, the Chicago Medical Society, and eminent physicians: H. Doyl Taylor, Joseph A. Sabatier, H. Thomas Ballantine, and James H. Sammons.

The trial took four whole years to even start after the initial lawsuit was filed. After two months, on January 29, 1981, the jury decided that the defendants had *not* violated any antitrust laws. The chiropractic profession, now much more organized, did not accept this defeat and sought to appeal. Wilk et al. versus the AMA went to court again on April 22, 1987. Five months of an uphill legal battle against the country's largest medical association led to a historic win for the chiropractic profession. US District Judge Susan Getzendanner had declared, "The American Medical Association (AMA) and its members participated in a conspiracy against chiropractors in violation of the nation's antitrust laws."

Special Communication ▄▄▄

IN THE UNITED STATES DISTRICT COURT
FOR THE NORTHERN DISTRICT OF ILLINOIS
EASTERN DIVISION

CHESTER A. WILK, et al.,   )
)
                    Plaintiffs,)
)
            v.   )   No. 76 C
)   3777
AMERICAN MEDICAL ASSOCIATION,)
et al.,   )
)
                    Defendants.)

PERMANENT INJUNCTION ORDER AGAINST AMA

Susan Getzendanner, District Judge

The court conducted a lengthy trial of this case in May and June of 1987 and on August 27, 1987, issued a 101 page opinion finding that the American Medical Association ("AMA") and its members participated in a conspiracy against chiropractors in violation of the nation's antitrust laws. Thereafter an opinion dated September 25, 1987 was substituted for the August 27, 1987 opinion. The question now before the court is the form of injunctive relief that the court will order.

A portion of the court injunction as published in the Journal of the American Medical Association. The full notice spanned just two pages.

The AMA petitioned to the US Supreme Court three separate times, all of which were denied. Judge Getzendanner submitted her final statements, which were published in the *Journal of the American Medical Association*. "The court has held that the conduct of the AMA and its members constituted a conspiracy in restraint of trade based on the following facts: the purpose of the boycott was to eliminate chiropractic; chiropractors are in competition with some medical physicians; the boycott had substantial anti-competitive effects; there were no pro-competitive effects of the boycott; and the plaintiffs were injured as a result of the conduct. These facts add up to a violation of the Sherman Act."[52]

Perhaps we have become so dependent on traditional health care and medicine because we were never offered any other approaches to healing. Maybe the *root cause* of today's health emergency can be found in the pivotal years between 1910 and 1976? Unfortunately, complex, multifaceted problems rarely have just one single origin. Using the foundational tool of root cause analysis (RCA), it's time to bring our attention to a deeper layer than recent history and politics. *Why* does our country maintain this dependence on medicine that permeates every facet of society, legislation, and education in our country? It is this one question, asked *repeatedly*, as Sakichi Toyoda did to usher in an era of innovation and transformation, that is the essence of RCA. That dedication to unearthing the true cause of the problem at hand is now our responsibility.

In any effective RCA, the first task is to *define the problem* clearly. Is the problem our *dependence* on medicine or the *outcomes* we receive because of this dependence?

---

[52]   Bart N. Green and Claire D. Johnson, ""Fighting Injustice: A Historical Review of the National Chiropractic Antitrust Committee,"" *Journal of Chiropractic Humanities* 26 (2019): 19–30.

CHAPTER 5

"HEALTH" CARE

"Marge, it takes two to lie. One to lie and one to listen."
—Homer Simpson

D R. Stephen Tower is a beloved orthopedic surgeon in the city of Anchorage, Alaska. Outside of his medical practice, he is a loving husband and an avid biker who regularly participates in one-hundred-mile races. But then his hip began to show signs of degenerative changes—pain and limited mobility. Dr. Tower was all too familiar with these symptoms. He was a prime candidate for having his hip replaced. In the groundbreaking Netflix documentary *Bleeding Edge*, Dr. Tower explained how the success of the hip replacement boils down to the materials used, of which the most common are ceramic-on-ceramic, ceramic-on-plastic, metal-on-plastic, and metal-on-metal. Dr. Tower, being the studious researcher he is, knew that the literature in medical-device journals demonstrated metal-on-metal (chrome cobalt) to be the best option for highly active individuals such as himself. Dr. Tower had no apprehensions about receiving this replacement, for he had successfully performed this same procedure on countless patients in the past. Within six weeks of his surgery, Dr. Tower was racing in two-hundred-mile events again, happy and content.

Within a year and a half of this routine procedure—the same procedure that millions of Americans go through each year—Dr. Tower began to show serious signs of physical and mental decline. "I developed a tremor in my nondominant hand," he recalled. That is, of course, especially problematic for a surgeon. His wife, Janice, remembers him complaining about terrible ringing in his ears as well as his decline in cognition. Dr. Tower was explaining himself over and over, repeating things, and finally, he experienced a psychological breakdown in a hotel room.

After the hotel-room incident, Dr. Tower began to investigate his own health crisis. After taking samples of his blood and urine, he discovered that the levels of cobalt in them were one hundred times what they should have been.[53] As soon as he could, he had his hip revised, removing the chrome cobalt implant and replacing it with a plastic-on-ceramic model. Luckily, Dr. Tower's story ends on a good note. Within a month of his new replacement, his symptoms were virtually nonexistent. That was it for Dr. Stephen Tower. After coming back from the brink of complete mental breakdown after the simple change of surgical material in his body, Dr. Tower began to test the blood and urine of all his patients who had the same kind of operation. He even teamed up with a diagnostic radiologist, Dr. Robert Bridges, to take positron emission tomography (PET) scans of the patients' brains, looking for signs of cognitive impairment likely caused by these replacements. Almost all his cobalt-replacement patients had positive findings confirmed

---

[53] *The Bleeding Edge*, directed by Kirby Dick (2018; Los Gatos, CA: Netflix), 99 min.

via PET scans. Dr. Bridges, after reviewing these different cases, couldn't help but wonder, "Is cobalt the new mercury poisoning? Are these people being relegated to the dustbin because they have what somebody misperceives as dementia? How many people have been misdiagnosed with a permanent disease process that has a *reversible* disease process?"

Although *some* hip manufacturers have indeed recalled *some* of their products because of nearby tissue rejection, these manufacturers still routinely recommend hip replacements that contain cobalt.

And this is where we are with our health care industry in 2025.

Modern medicine is not working. That's the problem. The heartbreaking problem of cobalt hip replacements and subsequent mental decline is just one example of the multitude of problems that exist within today's health care. Dr. Tower's story is only a symptom of a larger problem that is hiding in the shadows of our twisted health care system.

So now we return to a question we started out exploring: What is the true cost of modern medicine's orchestrated effort to create a monopoly on health? This myopic view on health care has taken a massive toll across the board, ranging from the actual quality of our health all the way down to the beliefs we are taught. We used *root cause analysis* to explore our first nagging question: Where does this dependency on modern medicine come from? Now we must use the same practice to dissect the actual reality of our health status. Nothing will ever change unless we genuinely acknowledge the most visible issue in our health care system: our actual quality of health—on both an individual and societal level.

Over one hundred years have passed since the publishing of the Flexner Report. In that interval, health care has gone through several evolutions. Hospitals and clinics multiplied manyfold as they became the primary location for all members of the public to receive care, not just the destitute. Between 1909 and 1932, the number of hospital beds in the country increased sixfold.[54]

The Hill-Burton Act of 1946, signed into law by President Truman, ensured that hospitals and other health facilities around the country had the necessary funding. In return, the government asked that those in the community who could not afford medical care be able to receive it at these community-based hospitals. This piece of legislation initiated a long series of debates among presidents and lawmakers over the issue of *how* citizens should be paying for medical care. President Franklin D. Roosevelt decided to not include health insurances in his Social Security Act. Although he wanted to, and was encouraged to, he feared it to be too controversial and feared that it would put his legislative agenda at risk. FDR's successors, Presidents Truman and Eisenhower, both attempted to carry on his legacy and enact federal health insurance but were rejected several times by Congress. Finally, in 1965, under President Lyndon B. Johnson, Medicare and Medicaid were enacted as Title XVIII and Title XIX of the Social Security Act. Medicare extended health coverage to almost all Americans aged sixty-five or older, and Medicaid provided health care services to those receiving welfare benefits.

---

[54]   Penn Nursing, "History of Hospitals," University of Pennsylvania School of Nursing, https://www.nursing.upenn.edu/nhhc/nurses-institutions-caring/history-of-hospitals/.

With every passing year, the health care scene rapidly changed, looking dramatically different every decade. More and more Americans had access to doctors and nurses around the clock. Pharmacies sprouted up across the country, and medicine was increasingly becoming the mainstream option for every citizen. But just as the *industry* of health care has evolved so too has the *quality* of our actual health changed.

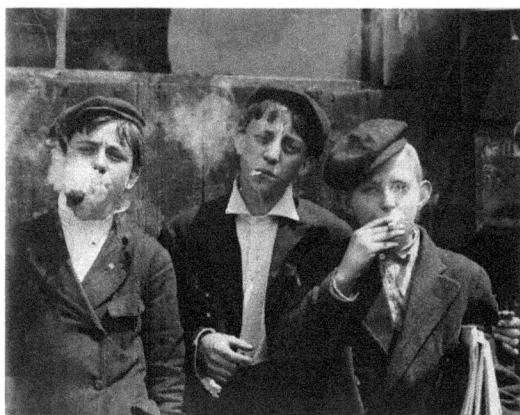

Young newsboys taking a break to smoke at
Skeeter's Branch, St. Louis, Missouri, 1910.

A hundred years ago, before widespread knowledge of hygiene, when children were regular consumers of cigarettes, one was more likely to die from infectious disease processes such as tuberculosis, pneumonia, or waterborne infections such as enteritis, than they were of today's chronic diseases such as cardiac disease or cancer.[55] Today, however, the overwhelming majority of people in the United States die of chronic illness. One-third of all deaths can be attributed to heart disease or

---

[55] Carolina Demography, "Mortality and Cause of Death, 1900 vs. 2010," June 16, 2014, https://carolinademography.cpc.unc.edu/2014/06/16/mortality-and-cause-of-death-1900-v-2010/.

stroke every year. Six hundred thousand people die each year from cancer. More than 38 million individuals have been diagnosed with diabetes, with another estimated 98million on the edge of developing full-blown diabetes.[56] Forty-two percent of adults in America are clinically obese, and child obesity is on the rise, putting them all at increased risk for cardiovascular disease, cancer, and diabetes. According to the Centers for Disease Control, 90 percent of US health care spending is for the treatment of chronic diseases. Recent estimates put US spending on health care at over $4 trillion each year. Here's what that looks like:

$$\$4,000,000,000,000$$

Over $14,000 spent on each person. And we still have 60 percent of US citizens living with chronic diseases?

Okay, so maybe on a smaller scale, individual health and medical care don't quite hit the mark in *creating* healthy individuals. And maybe that isn't the responsibility of the medical system. But what about on a much larger, more global scale? How does America's medical system fare when compared with those of similar countries? For $3 trillion a year, we should expect that the services we are all paying for get delivered effectively. By comparing each country's *amenable mortality*, we can see just how effective our treatment methods are. Amenable mortality refers to "rates of death considered *preventable* by timely and effective care." Data taken from the Healthcare

---

[56]   Centers for Disease Control and Prevention, "About Chronic Diseases," https://www.cdc.gov/chronicdisease/about/index.htm; National Cancer Institute, "Cancer Statistics," https://www.cancer.gov/about-cancer/understanding/statistics; Centers for Disease Control and Prevention, "National Diabetes Statistics Report," https://www.cdc.gov/diabetes/data/statistics-report/index.html.

Access and Quality Index show that the United States ranks *dead last* on that measure, having the highest rates of amenable mortality compared with similar countries

An additional way to assess a country's overall health and quality of care is its *all-cause mortality rate*—essentially, how many people die per one hundred thousand. Within the past hundred years, the US and other developed nations have seen mortality rates drop. However, as other nations (e.g., Belgium, Japan, Sweden, the UK) have had continual declines in mortality rates, the US has seemed to plateau. Data taken from the Kaiser Family Foundation reports that other countries have achieved significantly greater reductions in mortality rates for certain health conditions since 1980—up to 43 percent for some diseases—while in the United States, the reduction has been notably slower, with overall mortality decreasing by approximately 29 percent.[57] Maybe a 14 percent difference doesn't bother you. Perhaps you and your loved ones don't fall into the 60 percent category of Americans living with chronic illnesses and disabilities. Maybe you are not worried about the likelihood of needing surgery or emergency treatment like millions of people every day require. But what about the way life *starts* in America? Are we setting up our children and mothers for a healthy life?

You would logically assume that the more affluent countries have correspondingly lower maternal and child mortality rates, and in most cases, you would be correct. Sadly, the United States, despite having some of the world's most prestigious medical institutions with state-of-the-art technology, is an outlier when it comes to maternal and child mortality.

---

[57] Peterson-KFF Health System Tracker, "How Do U.S. Mortality Rates Compare?" May 19, 2022, https://www.healthsystemtracker.org/chart-collection/mortality-rates-u-s-compare-countries/.

For every 100,000 live births, countries similar to the US see around 5.3 deaths. The US sees 22.3 deaths per 100,000 (as of 2022).[58] That is a staggering statistic on its own and gets worse the deeper we look. Unfortunately, health care in the United States is intimately tied to race. Black women die during childbirth at a rate three times higher than white women. This is absolutely unacceptable. What are we getting wrong? Even the results of delivering babies are subpar when compared with other countries. Women in the United States who choose to deliver vaginally are much more likely to experience obstetric trauma, especially when instruments such as forceps are involved (Agency for Healthcare Research and Quality, "Obstetric Trauma during Vaginal Delivery")

The numbers aren't any better when we look at our children. *Health Affairs*, a leading international publication of health-policy research, recently published alarming data on the reality of child mortality in the United States. During the fifty years between 1961 and 2010, there have been tremendous advancements across all twenty listed nations in their child mortality rates. However, the journal reported that in the 1990s and into the 2000s, the US ranked lowest of all twenty nations in terms of child mortality rates. By the early 2000s, infants in the United States had a 74 percent higher risk of death, and kids aged one to nineteen had a 56 percent higher risk of death than nineteen other similar countries.[59]

---

[58]   Advisory Board, "Maternal Mortality Rates: The U.S. vs. Other Developed Nations," June 5, 2024, https://www.advisory.com/daily-briefing/2024/06/05/maternal-mortality.

[59]   Ellen Nolte and C. Martin McKee, "Measuring the Health of Nations: Updating an Earlier Analysis," *Health Affairs* 26, no. 1 (2007): 71–83.

Comparative Mortality Risk for Children and Infants
United States vs. 19 Industrialized Nations (1990s-2000s)

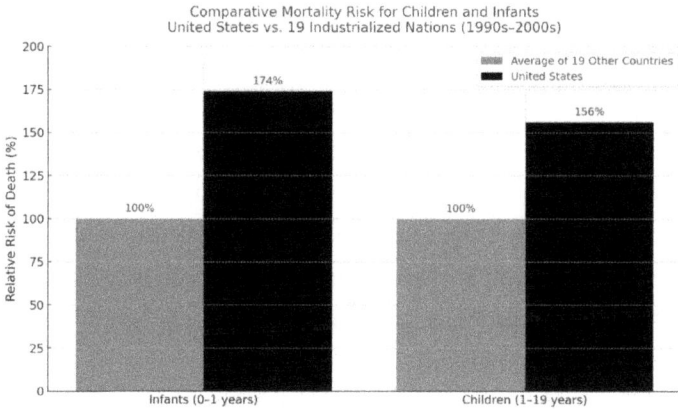

Source: Ellen Nolte and C. Martin McKee, "Measuring the Health of Nations: Updating an Earlier Analysis," Health Affairs 26, no. 1 (2007): 71-83.

Can we pause here for a moment to gain more focus?

The quality of our health, individual and collective, is a problem. The quality of the health care we are receiving is no longer optimal. The myopic, medicine-dependent approach to health care is no longer suited to our needs—and that too is a problem. Our health care system has evolved, or rather *devolved*, into a symptom-based society. This is a result of medical dependency that arose during a time of great infectious disease, when the symptoms were deadly and easily passed onto nearby individuals. Fortunately, because of advancements in sanitation, hygiene, and medical education, we have *evolved* beyond those devastating, infection-ridden decades and entered, instead, into an era of *chronic* illness. Why has medicine refused to evolve as well? We need immediate improvements in health care. It's nonnegotiable. We don't have to look very far ahead into the future to see what's coming.

Children and young adults are becoming increasingly sedentary. Screen time is just a way of life in our world now, and our human bodies were not designed to be sedentary organisms. Our brains aren't wired to be looking at a screen all day long. The chemical composition of soil is changing, causing less nutrient-rich food to grow, and the consumption of processed food is on the rise. So are conditions such as obesity, heart disease, and diabetes. From 2019 to 2020, pediatric hospitalization rates for type 2 diabetes *doubled*.[60]

The way we care for our health in this country must change. If we wish to change the outcomes, we *must* critically analyze our health practices. Using our root cause analysis tools, we must look deeper than our current outcome. We must ask ourselves what behaviors, or practices, drove us here? Einstein said it best: "Insanity is doing the same thing over and over and expecting different results." Unfortunately, most of the practices our system uses have become habitual, no longer serving our best interests, and in too many areas they seem to have become unconscious. Habits are a son of bitch, aren't they?

It's easy to want to reject the status quo when we see all of these shocking statistics about mortality rates and chronic illnesses. We might even want to march down the street waving signs and calling out elected leaders in charge of making reforms. But unless we understand the specific *practices* happening every day in our country, then nothing will ever change. Perhaps if more people were made aware of the daily goings-on in the mainstream medical system, then less emphasis would

---

[60] Hagar Shimony et al., "Pediatric Diabetes Mellitus Hospitalizations and COVID-19 Pandemic Response Measures," *Diabetes Research and Clinical Practice* 207 (January 2024): 111060.

be placed on "who foots the bill" and more on the quality of the care received.

A few specific practices that our health care system has taken on are directly contributing to the atrocious quality of your health and your children's health. Dozens of medical, health, and legal experts agree that there are three main areas of health care behaviors we need to address if we expect anything to positively change. First on the list is the pharmaceutical industry's marketing efforts that are corrupting honest, hard-working family doctors. Then there are that same industry's incomplete, nontransparent research methods. Finally, the experts have identified problems with the fast-track method by which medical technology is approved for human use. These are not the only cancerous habits our medical system upholds; they are just the most prominent ones.

CHAPTER 6

SICK MEDICINE

"It didn't occur to me until later that there's another truth, very simple: greed in a good cause is still greed."

—Stephen King

I T MAY NOT seem outrageous that pharmaceutical companies are allowed to openly advertise drugs in this country. But when you consider the fact that the United States is one of only two countries on Earth in which they are allowed to do so, well, things start to appear a little less cut and dried. When it comes to the marketing efforts of the various pharmaceutical companies, there is little, if any, real consideration for patient care. Take opioids, for example. In 2015, nearly 45 percent of all opioid-related deaths involved a prescription opioid.[61] Today's headlines frequently mention fentanyl. According to the Centers for Disease Control and Prevention, fentanyl is a synthetic opioid that is up to fifty times stronger than heroin

---

[61] Guy GP Jr. et al., "Vital Signs: Changes in Opioid Prescribing in the United States, 2006–2015," *MMWR Morbidity and Mortality Weekly Report* 66 (2017): 697–704.

and a hundred times stronger than morphine. Fentanyl use has skyrocketed in the past several years and claims the life of one individual every 8.5 minutes in the United States.[62] Prescribed brand-name opioids such as OxyContin are often the first opioids people are introduced to before fentanyl.

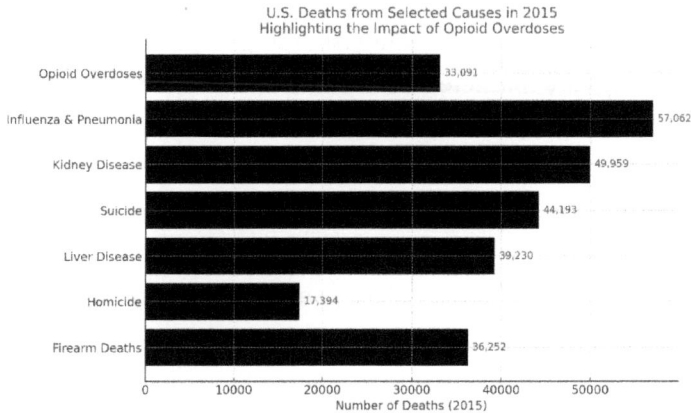

U.S. Deaths from Selected Causes in 2015
Highlighting the Impact of Opioid Overdoses

Cause	Deaths
Opioid Overdoses	33,091
Influenza & Pneumonia	57,062
Kidney Disease	49,959
Suicide	44,193
Liver Disease	39,230
Homicide	17,394
Firearm Deaths	36,252

Number of Deaths (2015)

*

Source: CDC National Vital Statistics Reports, 2015; Opioid data from CDC MMWR, 2016

During the height of the opioid epidemic, more than 130 people were dying every day; 33,000 people died of opioid overdoses in 2015.[63] In 2017, the epidemic was declared a national health emergency. Detailed accounts have appeared of the infamous Sackler family and Purdue Pharma: a book, *The Empire of Pain*; a documentary, *All the Beauty and the Bloodshed*; and even a hit television series, *Dopesick*, have brought much needed attention to the issue of opioids. By now most people

---

[62]   National Institute on Drug Abuse, "Overdose Death Rates," *National Institutes of Health*, https://nida.nih.gov/research-topics/trends-statistics/overdose-death-rates.

[63]   Centers for Disease Control and Prevention, "Drug and Opioid-Involved Overdose Deaths, 2013–2017," *MMWR* 67, no. 12 (2018): 1419–1427.

have some level of awareness of the dangers of opioid drugs. Has the United States made a concerted effort to counteract this massive health emergency? To a degree. It is true that since 2010 the country has seen a reduction in prescribing rate, but, sadly, as of 2015 it is still three times higher than in 1999.[64] Until very recently, consumers (possibly including you and your loved ones) had no understanding of how these danger-ous drugs are marketed. And so researchers from the Boston University School of Medicine set out to truly understand the association between direct-to-physician marketing of opioid products by pharmaceutical companies and the subsequent mortality from prescription opioid overdoses. Posting their findings in the *Journal of the American Medical Association* (*JAMA*), this team, led by Dr. Scott E. Hadland, carefully stud-ied every single county in the United States between August 1, 2013, and December 31, 2015, analyzing opioid marketing efforts, payments to physicians, opioid prescription rates, and mortality related to overdosing on opioids. Here is their report: "We extracted every transfer of value ('payment') in marketing from a pharmaceutical company to a physician as mandated by the recent Physician Payments Sunshine Act. Each entry in the Open Payments database includes the monetary value of the payment in dollars, the medication(s) being marketed, the type of marketing (i.e., meals, travel costs, speaking fees, honoraria, consulting fees, or educational costs), and the physi-cian practice location."[65]

[64]   Abay Asfaw et al., "Work Injuries and Opioid Prescriptions," *J Occup Environ Med* 64, no. 12 (2022): e823–e832.

[65]   John Trecki, "A Perspective Regarding the Current State of the Opioid Epidemic," *JAMA Network Open* 2, no. 1 (2019): e187104.

We now know that between 2013 and 2015, one in twelve US physicians received opioid-related marketing. If you took that same set of data and applied it to only doctors who practiced family medicine, the number is closer to one in five.[66] We now know that there were 434,754 payments totaling $39.7 million in non-research-based opioid marketing. And what did all of this marketing lead to throughout the various counties across the country? Increased opioid prescribing… and increased opioid overdoses.

The opioid crisis has garnered substantial attention and focus from governmental agencies, nonprofit organizations, celebrities, and advocacy groups, as it most certainly should. However, this gross behavior of direct-to-physician marketing is not exclusive to the opioid manufacturers. Across the board, doctors who received money from pharmaceutical companies (in any form) prescribed more of their drug. The investigative journalistic publishing outlet *Propublica* has outlined how this pharma marketing is pervasive among doctors across the board, not just regarding opioids. Primarily using data from the Medicare Part D drug program, they studied the fifty most-prescribed brand-name drugs in Medicare for which drugmakers had made payments to doctors in 2016, including treatments for diabetes, asthma, high cholesterol, hypertension, and glaucoma.[67]

Linzess is commonly prescribed for patients dealing with irritable bowel syndrome. From 2014 to 2018, the drug's manu-

---

[66] Scott E. Hadland et al., "Physician Prescribing and Stimulant Misuse," *NIH HEAL Initiative*, July 2021, https://heal.nih.gov/files/2021-07/physician-prescribing-stimulant-misuse-hadland.pdf.

[67] Ornstein and Jones, "Doctors Prescribe More of a Drug If They Receive Money"

facturers, Allergan and Ironwood, spent nearly $29 million on payments to doctors related to Linzess.[68] These payments, similar to those for opioids, were largely in the form of expensive dining events and promotional speaking fees. Doctors who received payments related to Linzess in 2016 wrote 45 percent more prescriptions for the drug than doctors who received no payments. Or how about the fact that doctors who received payments for the overactive-bladder drug Myrbetriq wrote 64 percent more prescriptions for the drug than doctors who did not receive payment? And what about the chronic dry eye medication Restasis? The doctors who received kickbacks for this drug prescribed it at a rate 141 percent higher than their unpaid colleagues.[69] What is going on? Remember, the majority of this data came from studying Medicare drug programs. The financial burden of our overmedicated senior population began to accumulate to the point that the Department of Health and Human Services issued a report in which they stated, "The Medicare program, through its Part D plans, spent almost $9 billion on brand-name drugs when therapeutically equivalent generics were available. If these prescriptions were instead dispensed as generics, the Part D program and its beneficiaries would have saved almost $3 billion."[70]

[68]   Charles Ornstein and Ryann Grochowski Jones, "Doctors Prescribe More of a Drug If They Receive Money from a Pharma Company Tied to It," *ProPublica*, March 17, 2016.

[69]   Charles Ornstein and Ryann Grochowski Jones, "Doctors Prescribe More of a Drug If They Receive Money from a Pharma Company Tied to It," *ProPublica*, March 17, 2016.

[70]   U.S. Department of Health and Human Services, *Savings Available Under Full Generic Substitution of Multiple Source Brand Drugs in Medicare Part D*, July 23, 2018.

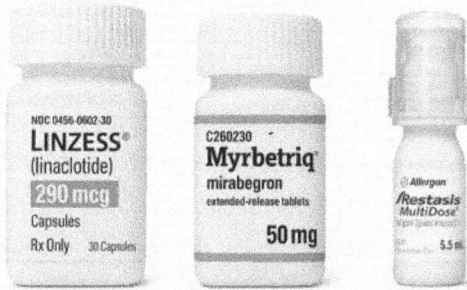

| 45% More prescriptions | 64% More Prescriptions | 141% More Prescriptions |

Between a four-year span, drug manufacturers spent $29 million on payments to doctors related to Linzess.

Behaviors drive outcomes. We all agree that our collective health is suffering, the quality of our health care is declining, and the future is not looking bright for our children. This is not new information, nor is it surprising, but things will never change unless we address at least some of the habits that lead us to these kinds of outcomes. The amount of money that is circulating throughout the medical health care industry is focused on profit, not on the well-being of patients. How long are we going to accept the fact that pharmaceutical representatives, who are not medically trained, can easily influence the decision-making process of a medical doctor? Wouldn't you want to know if your children's family physician had recently been taken to a luxurious dinner by Purdue Pharma, Merck, or any other drug manufacturing company? How can we be expected to trust the objectivity of our medical providers when financial influence runs so rampant?

Some people would argue that the more money a pharmaceutical company spends on marketing, the more people they can reach with their drug and, by doing so, help them. Let's talk about that for a moment. Let's set aside the shady methods by which pharmaceutical companies market their drugs and focus instead on what should matter the most: the science. Who cares how much money a private company spends on advertising its drugs if the drug itself is of high quality and caliber, right?

Research posted in *The British Medical Journal* investigated the quality of drugs entering the market. Authors Donald Light, a prestigious medical sociologist, and Joel Lexchin, the author of over 160 peer-reviewed publications, wanted to know the kind of therapeutic advances being made by the pharmaceutical industry. Every year, more and more *new drugs* appear on the market. But are these new drugs that much different from the older, more generic ones, with *different* being defined as "having an active ingredient that has never been marketed in any form"? And more important than that, are these drugs that much *better* for the patient? Light and Lexchin sampled three different periods of time: 1978–1989, 1974–1994, and the mid-1990s onward. Between 1978 and 1989, the FDA approved 218 drugs for use. Only 15.6 percent of those drugs showed important therapeutic gains when compared with other drugs in the same "family." Between 1974 and 1994, all internationally marketed drugs were analyzed. Only 11 percent were "therapeutically and pharmacologically innovative." Of all new drugs distributed since the mid-1990s, 85 to 90 percent have provided "few or no clinical advantages for patients."[71]

This stunning lack of genuine scientific advancement becomes even more concerning when we consider how these drug companies have been prioritizing their funds. According

---

[71] Donald W. Light and Joel R. Lexchin, "Pharmaceutical Research and Development: What Do We Get for All That Money?" *BMJ* 345 (2012): e4348.

to the National Science Foundation and government reports, pharmaceutical companies have been spending around 1.3 percent of their revenues on research to discover innovative new molecules for their drugs. Independent analysis estimates that these companies spent around 25 percent of their revenues on promoting their drugs.[72]

Regarding the infamous Flexner Report, Abraham Flexner's intention was to improve the standards and guidelines within medical education. Science and technological advancement were to bring us out of the Wild West that was our health care. Science—or perhaps we should say "medical science"—was to be the gold standard, as the Flexner Report was no doubt instrumental in stamping out naturopaths and homeopaths. And it gave chiropractors and osteopaths an uphill battle for recognition and acceptance, all in the name of advancement. Less than one hundred years later, we are faced with a population that has a growing dependence on an industry that isn't even dedicated to putting its own funds into better research and therapeutic gains.

When Sakichi Toyoda's intricate looms malfunctioned or produced subpar fabric, he and his team would take the entire machine apart. Piece by piece, they would examine all facets of it to understand the true root cause of the malfunction, which was almost always human error. When we look at how these pharmaceutical companies conduct research compared with how they conduct their marketing, it does not take a scientist to understand why these drugs are so ineffective, addicting, and dangerous. The way in which pharmaceutical research is

---

[72]   Marc-André Gagnon and Joel Lexchin, "The Cost of Pushing Pills: A New Estimate of Pharmaceutical Promotion Expenditures in the United States," *PLoS Medicine* 5, no. 1 (2008): e1.

conducted is a lot like how children clean their rooms in an attempt to be allowed to go to a friend's house—hastily, incompletely, with a whole lot of questionable items stuffed into the closet. Let's unpack that closet a little bit.

There is no clean, pretty way to unpack the mess that is pharmaceutical research, so we might as well get down and dirty with it. For drugs to make it to the public, they must go through many rounds of testing and several different phases of clinical trials. And these trials are wildly expensive to run. Given the fact that brand-name drugs are where companies make the bulk of their income, there is a lot of pressure to get their expensive drug to consumers. A 2014 study published in *Nature Biotechnology* found that only about 34 percent of these trials make it to the final phase of testing, further turning up the pressure these companies are under to have positive outcomes.

Currently, pharmaceutical companies are allowed to fund and design their own trials, and unbeknownst to most people, they choose the trial results that get handed over to journals and peer reviewers. (Read that over as many times as you need to.) This is bad science. *The Washington Post* reported on a sampling of seventy-three original research articles from *The New England Journal of Medicine*, the most prestigious and cited medical journal in the world. Of these seventy-three studies, sixty had been funded by a pharmaceutical company, fifty included the pharmaceutical company's employees among the authors, and the lead researchers of thirty-seven studies had accepted financial compensation from the drug company.[73]

When it comes to *objectivity*—a cornerstone of science—the question of who pays for the research is critical. The pub-

---

[73]   *The Washington Post*, "Analysis of Research Articles Published in the New England Journal of Medicine."

licly funded National Institutes of Health (NIH), which is responsible for biomedical and public health research, has been funding less and less research each year, allowing for pharmaceutical companies to foot the bill themselves. In 2014, the pharmaceutical industry paid for 6,550 trials, while NIH funded 1,048. These startling data were published in *JAMA*.[74]

Public Citizen is a nonprofit, progressive consumer-rights advocacy group. Its director, Dr. Michael Carome, is an expert on issues of drug and medical-device safety, pharmacy compounding, US Food and Drug Administration oversight, health care policy, and the protection of human research subjects. When it comes to publication bias, he says there are significant issues within the pharmaceutical industry. Dr. Carome has publicly stated: "The decision to publish the results of a study on a particular drug lies entirely with the study's investigators, including pharmaceutical companies who conduct and fund clinical trials testing their drug products. The medical literature is thus a partial, and often biased, sample of all medical evidence."[75]

Have you ever heard of the popular antiflu drug Tamiflu? Roche, which manufactures the drug, advertised it as an effective way to fight the flu and its symptoms. Cochrane is a British international charitable organization formed to organize medical research to evaluate the safety and effectiveness of different drugs and procedures. In 2014, this organization evaluated Tamiflu. After carefully combing through seventy clinical trials and accumulating more than one hundred thou-

---

[74] Stephan Ehrhardt, Lawrence J. Appel, and Curtis L. Meinert, "Trends in National Institutes of Health Funding for Clinical Trials Registered in ClinicalTrials.gov," *JAMA* 314, no. 23 (2015): 2566–2567.

[75] *Drugwatch*, "Big Pharma & Clinical Trials: Funding, Influence & Corruption."

sand pages of unpublished data, they found that Tamiflu had little to no benefit in preventing the flu or shortening the duration of flu symptoms.[76]

The amount of tolerance we allow for these kinds of practices not only leads to bad science and poor health, but it also leads to unnecessary death and suffering. One of the most notorious examples is the Vioxx scandal involving Merck & Co. and *The New England Journal of Medicine.* John Abramson served as a family physician for twenty-two years and also worked for ten years, from 2004 to 2014, as an expert for lawyers suing pharmaceutical companies. He has donated his time and expertise to the FBI and Department of Justice on numerous occasions and currently is on faculty at Harvard Medical School, where he teaches health care policy. John Abramson understands (like no other) the world of pharmaceutical politics and practices and has publicly detailed their criminal actions in best-selling books. Abramson pinpointed the heart of the issue with regard to the pharmaceutical industry when he said, "It is Big Pharma that funds most clinical trials and therefore controls the research agenda, withholds the real data from those trials as corporate secrets, and shapes most of the information relied upon by health care professionals." Such was the story of Vioxx, a case in which Abramson played a key role in investigation and litigation.[77]

---

[76]   Tom Jefferson et al., "Neuraminidase Inhibitors for Preventing and Treating Influenza in Adults and Children," *Cochrane Database of Systematic Reviews* 2014, no. 4 (2014): CD008965.

[77]   John Abramson, *Sickening: How Big Pharma Broke American Health Care and How We Can Repair It* (Boston: Mariner Books, 2022).

"Between 20-25 million Americans had taken Vioxx and between 40,000 and 60,000 Americans had died from the cardiovascular consequences of Vioxx. It was no more effective at treating aches and pains than other nonsteroidal anti-inflammatories."

—John Abramson

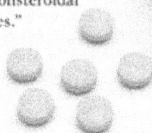

Vioxx is a nonsteroidal anti-inflammatory drug used to treat the pain associated with osteo- and rheumatoid arthritis, migraines, and menstrual cramping. Marketed by Merck & Co, Vioxx was said to be superior to other pain medications such as Naproxen, because Vioxx had a much lower risk of gastrointestinal complications. And that is what was published in *The New England Journal of Medicine* (*NEJM*) in an article sponsored by the drug's manufacturer, Merck, stating, "Vioxx is a better option for reducing the risk of GI problems."[78]

This article was followed by another Vioxx article, this time admitting to the cardiovascular problems caused by the arthritis drug. The authors of the second article said that the cardiovascular problems may not be clinically significant since there were "only 70 events," and such a small number of events is subject to statistical variation. This is where John Abramson decided to involve himself. Remember, the only reason this drug was being sold was the claim that it was safer for the patient's GI tract, and there were only fifty-three serious GI

---

[78]   Claire Bombardier et al., "Comparison of Upper Gastrointestinal Toxicity of Rofecoxib and Naproxen in Patients with Rheumatoid Arthritis," *The New England Journal of Medicine* 343, no. 21 (2000): 1520–1528.

events listed in this review article published by the *NEJM*. Dr. Abramson knew that the seventy adverse cardiovascular reactions could in no way be chance, as the drug's manufacturers were claiming. Two weeks after this article came out, *JAMA*, another major prestigious journal, published a Vioxx article that included a footnote that linked to an FDA website with the data showing how fraudulent Merck had been about Vioxx. Under much pressure, Merck put out an additional study on Vioxx, and this time the data it included about Vioxx showed that the risk of stroke or heart attack had doubled.[79] Abramson said, "Between 20–25 million Americans had taken Vioxx and between 40,000 and 60,000 Americans had died from the cardiovascular consequences of Vioxx. It was no more effective at treating aches and pains than other nonsteroidal anti-inflammatories."[80]

So what were the consequences of all this deceit and fraud? It ended up with 27,000 plaintiffs in the litigation, and they were awarded $4.7 billion for their injuries and suffering. In the four years Vioxx was on the market, Merck sold $12 billion worth. No one went to jail. What you would like to hear, of course, is that this scandal was a rare event. Unfortunately, experts on this topic would say otherwise. Abramson wrote: "Medical journals are caught up in this. The journals tolerate peer reviewers not getting the data. The peer reviewers don't get the data. The medical journal editors don't get the data, so they don't really know what is true. They say these articles are peer-reviewed, but they don't get the data. This goes from

---

[79]   *CBS News*, "Timeline of Vioxx-Related Events."

[80]   UNC School of Medicine, "Medicine Grand Rounds: Dr. John Abramson Presents 'Why We Can't Trust the Evidence in Evidence-Based Medicine.'"

the *New England Journal* to *JAMA* on down. They don't get the data."[81]

Abramson has exposed one of the best-kept secrets within the pharmaceutical industry: lack of *peer review*—two words that, when attached to a statement, claim, or publication, add instant legitimacy and credibility. The peer review process *is supposed to* assess the quality and validity of a manuscript before its publication in a journal. Independent reviewers critique the data they have been given and provide honest feedback on the quality of the science. They also make recommendations to the publisher as to whether the article should be published.

What is the reason for the secrecy the pharmaceutical industry enjoys around this process? Peer reviewers responsible for assessing these companies' accuracy and scientific integrity do not even have access to complete data and must rely on corporate-influenced summaries. Same for the experts who write the clinical practice guidelines that define our standards of care. They don't get the complete data! They have to make recommendations on manuscripts summarizing the data from the trials. That is how Vioxx can be publicized in places such as *The New England Journal of Medicine*, look amazing to doctors, get prescribed at high rates…and injure and kill thousands. But hey, as long as the science was peer-reviewed, right?

Take a deep breath. We are almost done with the messy part.

We have just acknowledged two significant areas of concern when it comes to how our country practices health care. The promotion and marketing of pharmaceutical products costs exponentially more than their research efforts and to

---

[81]   *Corporate Crime Reporter*, "John Abramson on How Big Pharma Broke American Health Care."

a large degree corrupts the clinical objectivity of genuine, hardworking doctors. That must end. We are overmedicated compared with people from all other countries, but we aren't healthier for it. Infectious disease has been on the decline for decades, but chronic illness has been steadily rising. We must promote health care that addresses *that* situation.

Does this mean that there should be a world in which pharmaceutical medication does not exist? Of course not; medication saves lives every day, and thousands of hardworking biotech students, researchers, and doctors dedicate their lives to this process. Unfortunately, they exist in a world that prioritizes profits over clinical excellence. Money corrupts all institutions, and it's sadly clear that the research and publishing institutions are not immune. If we wish to allow transparent and genuine science to prosper, we must reform the process by which data is reviewed—no more haphazard summaries written by pharmaceutical employees and handed to prestigious academic journals. We need to have more publicly funded trials. We need to get money out of science, or at the very least, stop persecuting those who are questioning the authority of these institutions putting out bad science into this world.

There is one more malignant practice the medical industry allows to thrive that is detrimental to both the scientific process and the health and well-being of everyday people. It's the process by which medical technology is authorized for human use. Tongue depressors, medical gauze, insulin pumps, and surgical mesh all fall under the category of "medical technology." Some medical technology is extremely low risk, such as medical gloves. On the other hand, devices such as pacemakers and joint replacements are much higher-risk medical technologies. If you think that the process by which pharmaceuticals get approved is too fast and unregulated, let's talk about medical technology in the United States.

There are two paths by which medical devices can gain FDA approval for use. The original method, and the one Congress had intended for *all* devices to gain approval, is through the premarket approval (PMA) process. The PMA is like the pharmaceutical drug journey. The medical device must be extensively studied in human clinical trials, detailed and comprehensive data must be recorded, and the data must be submitted to FDA scientists to determine safety and effectiveness. The MedTech market, which as of 2020 was valued at approximately $456.9 billion, has been very vocal in its complaints about the premarket approval process.[82] The industry claims that this process of research and development can become increasingly expensive and repetitive considering that every year there are advancements and updates on the various kinds of technology and devices that are currently approved on the market, and taking the same device through lengthy research trials every time there is an update may be unwarranted.

And so Congress passed the second path by which medical devices can gain FDA approval, the 510(k) process. This way, the only thing the manufacturers have to prove is that their device (contraceptives, pacemakers, joint replacements) is "substantially equivalent" to another device that is already on the market.[83] The FDA considers devices to be equivalent based on two criteria:

1. It has the same intended use as the predicate device and the same technological characteristics.

---

[82] *AlphaSense, Medtech and Medical Device Outlook for 2024 & Beyond.*

[83] U.S. Food and Drug Administration, *510(k) Premarket Notification Program: Guidance for Industry and FDA Staff.*

2. It has the same intended use as the predicate device, has different technological characteristics, does not raise new questions of safety and effectiveness, and the applicant can show that the device is at least as safe and effective as the marketed device.

If the above criteria have been met, the device in question is no longer put through safety and efficacy trials, saving the manufacturers both time and money. All the 510(k) process guarantees is that the new device coming out is similar enough to the predicate device—another instance in which profit is prioritized over the well-being of human beings. Research shows that devices cleared through the 510(k) process are 11.5 times more likely to be recalled than devices that had more research and testing trials. In 2016, over 180 million devices were recalled.[84] This was the case for poor Dr. Stephen Tower and his metal-on-metal hip replacement.

At this point of our journey, as we turn over all these stones in our health care system, would you even be surprised to hear that between 95 and 98 percent of all medical devices on sale in the United States have been cleared through the abysmal 510(k) process?[85] Here is the worst part about all of this: even if a predicate device were taken off the market because of failing safety and efficacy characteristics, devices currently going through the 510(k) process can still be approved if they are

---

[84] Matthew D. Somberg et al., "Analysis of FDA-Approved Orthopaedic Devices and Their Recalls," *The Journal of Bone & Joint Surgery* 98, no. 6 (2016): 517–524; *PR Newswire*, "High-Price Device Race to Innovate: Medical Devices Fuels More Product Recalls," February 8, 2017.

[85] *Drugwatch*, "FDA 510(k) Clearance Process: How Medical Devices Reach the Market."

deemed to be "substantially equivalent." This is not a lie or a sick joke.

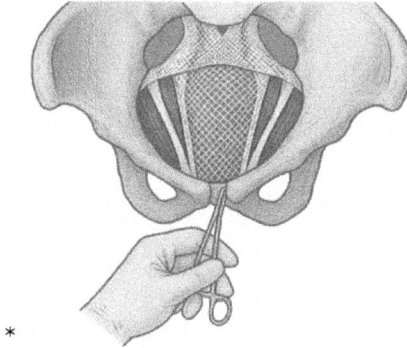

Illustration of transvaginal mesh.

An unfortunate example of this all-too-common malpractice is the transvaginal mesh, such as ProteGen, that is used for a variety of purposes including prolapse injuries or urinary incontinence. The FDA cleared the first mesh to be used for urinary incontinence in 1996. Three years later, after countless injuries and lawsuits, Boston Scientific, the maker of ProteGen, recalled the device. In the few years that ProteGen was on the market, several other mesh devices were approved through the 510(k) process using this about-to-be-recalled mesh as their reference.[86] Many other manufacturers still use the ProteGen sling as a predicate device and model theirs after it. Diana Zuckerman, president of the National Center for Health Research, has said, "The 510(k) program is the weakest and most nonsensical program in the FDA."

And yet every day, the FDA clears medical devices this way. Devices that are surgically inserted into your family and friends, with criminally low levels of oversight or regulation.

---

[86]   Panish Shea & Boyle LLP, "510(k) Loophole in Medical Device Cases."

Every day, pharmaceutical companies, despite decades of research showing the dangers of aggressive marketing, still go forth into your communities and present incomplete research to family physicians who are just trying to do what's best for you and your children.

What chance does the American public have when internationally revered journals such as *JAMA* and the *NEJM* don't even properly regulate the science being published in their journals? These are journal articles that primary care doctors depend on when it comes to staying up to date on the changing science. Articles that could quite literally save a life. What happens when the families of those who have died because of these dangerous drugs decide to take action? These multibillion-dollar companies are required only to pay fines and recall certain products. No one sees jail time, despite criminal and fraudulent actions, let alone a complete disregard for the scientific process.

Every day, a news article gets published on the failing quality of health in our country. Physical and mental health are declining. Surgery and medication rates are increasing. Medical debt is increasing. Things are not looking good. But why are we not considering, at least at a national level, that perhaps our poor outcomes are a manifestation of our profit-driven "health" care practices? That *maybe* all of this utter lack of real research, transparency, and accountability is linked to statistics we are seeing every day.

Is this the fault of any one person or industry? Of course not. But everything we have just talked about has been our status quo for way too long. This acceptance is now a part of our unconscious, automatic behavior. And like most behaviors, it is learned or, in this case, taught. This brings us to the last part of the problem with our current, traditional medical care system: belief systems. If we wish to honor Sakichi Toyoda's brilliant method of problem-solving, we must take our analysis as deep as it can possibly go. We can sit back and point the finger at the pharmaceutical companies that prioritize profits over people; we can blame regulatory agencies such as the FDA for allowing all of this bad science to go forth; we can fault prestigious medical journals for not truly critiquing data they publish—as well we should. However, to a certain extent, that's just business. It is now clear that these are *industries* hiding under the guise of health care. They have manipulated medical doctors and medical schools into thinking and practicing homogenously.

If this version of health care is not your ideal way of keeping yourself and your children safe and thriving, if you're tired of paying exorbitant amounts of money on health insurance and never receiving quality care, if you think there is a better way than what we have been told, then *you* can play a pivotal role in changing this system. If we wish to reject the status quo, *we* have to address our belief systems about health that enable these kinds of companies and industries to take advantage of us in this way.

CHAPTER 7

FEELINGS DO MATTER!

"If you change the belief first, changing the action is easier."
—Peter McWilliams

IMAGINE AN ELEPHANT and its rider setting out on their path. The rider may have the necessary coordinates of their journey, experience with the terrain, and the intellectual know-how. But all of this is of no consequence unless the elephant is on board with the rider. An African savanna elephant can weigh up to thirteen thousand pounds. However, let's not forget the importance of the rider. Let's assume that the region has poachers roaming around or perhaps other nearby dangers. An elephant out in the wild by itself can get into serious trouble. The rider knows where danger is and where camp is and can expertly guide the elephant to safety. Symbiosis is not just encouraged, it is required in this scenario.

In his book *The Happiness Hypothesis*, social psychologist Jonathan Haidt breaks down the relationship between our emotional side (the Elephant), and our analytical, rational side (its Rider). Haidt says, "Anytime the six-ton Elephant and the Rider disagree about which direction to go, the Rider is going to lose. He's completely overmatched."[87]

This is a strategy that companies and industries have expertly integrated into modern health care, and it started over one hundred years ago. Consider the infectious diseases (e.g., cholera, tuberculosis, smallpox) that were engulfing entire communities before major breakthroughs in sanitation and medicine. It was an incredibly emotional period, during which children were needlessly dying. With the invention of penicillin in 1928, millions of lives were saved. Fast forward to today. Emotion is just as present, if not more so, in health care and the corporate corruption of health care. Have you ever sat through a pharmaceutical advertisement in its entirety? It's always an individual in clear distress. A mother who is unable to sit through her child's school play because of IBS. An older man who can't lift his grandkids on account of his arthritic pain. A hardworking professional woman bedridden with migraines, unable to work. And then suddenly a pharmaceutical product (with questionable research data) appears on screen, the music changes to an upbeat tempo, and we can see all of those sad individuals now actually enjoying their lives with friends, families, and work. Oh, look, the older couple is kayaking! Never mind the side effects that include gastrointestinal bleeding and, at worst, death. Surely those are exceedingly *rare* and would *not* happen to *me*. Note this statistic: since 2018, television viewers have been exposed to half a million commercials—187 differ-

---

[87]   Jonathan Haidt, *The Happiness Hypothesis: Finding Modern Truth in Ancient Wisdom* (New York: Basic Books, 2006).

ent ads for seventy different pharmaceutical drugs.[88] How do you think child and adolescent minds respond to this kind of expert marketing? This is what modern medicine or should we say modern companies and industries under the guise of "medicine" are doing to our country: complete manipulation of how we think about health. We have become a *symptom-based society!*

OK, but what does that really mean? Consider a child or an average American adult with limited health knowledge. Many Americans receive most of their information and news from printed, televised, or internet media outlets. We know that all these sources of news and entertainment are heavily saturated with pharmaceutical advertising detailing symptoms for various illnesses and conditions. So right away, the average American is already associating the presence of symptoms with poor health. This is emotional conditioning.

We also know that health insurance in this country is atrocious. Millions are without it, which sadly causes those people to avoid proactive health care until there is a health crisis. For others, it is not a matter of finances. Because of emotional conditioning, people genuinely believe that the simple absence of symptoms is all they need to have a clean bill of health, and so action does not need to be taken until symptoms start to express themselves. This way of thinking could not be more wrong.

In 1948, the World Health Organization (WHO) came out with a comprehensive definition of health, describing it as a "state of complete physical, mental and social well-being

---

[88] *BioPharma Dive*, "Pharma Ad DTC Marketing: $2.8 Billion Spent on TV in 2018," last modified October 15, 2018, https://www.bio-pharmadive.com/news/pharma-ad-dtc-marketing-2018-spend-TV-congress/533319/.

and not merely the absence of disease or infirmity." According to the WHO, health is more than just "not feeling ill." After decades of research, we know that an essential foundation of mental health is good physical health. Aerobic exercise, gut microbiome, and systemic inflammation are all examples of physical health factors with effects on mental well-being. Expanding on this definition of health, we can comfortably say that even if someone tests positive for the seasonal flu (influenza), that person may not actually be unhealthy if tests also show perfect blood pressure, healthy blood sugar levels, strong physical capabilities, and so on. To label that individual as unhealthy just because of a viral infection isn't fair. Conversely, take an average American male in his fifties. On the outside, he may appear to be in good physical health, with no apparent illness or disabilities. We wouldn't be able to know the dangerously high levels of triglycerides and arteriosclerosis buildup until a potentially critical crisis occurs, such as a heart attack. Health is so much more than the presence or absence of symptoms.

This is possibly the biggest problem in our culture's approach to health care. *Beliefs matter.* What we believe dictates the behaviors we have, which lead to the outcomes we receive. These symptom-driven beliefs are not always black-and-white. They are subtle and nuanced. They dominate all aspects of our culture. Let's talk about social norms for a moment.

Columbia sociology professor Diane Vaughan has extensively studied problem-solving and management from a sociological perspective. In her critically acclaimed book, *The Challenger Launch Decision*, she explored the concept of *normalization of deviance* and how it specifically applies to that tragic accident. Vaughan pointed to the overwhelming lack of concern around the *Challenger*'s rocket-booster seals, despite multiple warnings.[89] Ignoring the warning signs of potential danger had become a habit on the part of NASA managers. And in the case of the *Challenger* shuttle, that habit ended in death and tragedy for an entire nation.

So what happens when habits such as ignoring warning signs spill over to other facets of society, particularly around health and illness? Social normalization of deviance means that people have become so used to poor health and overmedicating that we no longer see those problems as *problems*. We actually believe them to be normal. And when we see our behaviors and health as normal, why would we ever do anything different? We have millions of people in this country who only ever act on their health when a symptom is present. And what have most people been conditioned to do about their symptoms? Suppress them with medication. Do you have a migraine? Just take Excedrin. Suffer from heartburn? Omeprazole. Are you considered to be prediabetic? Metformin to the rescue.

Of course, medications are not evil, and people should not have to suffer needlessly. However, this symptom-based cycle pretty much never addresses the *root causes* of illness and disease. Modern medicine has expertly taken control of our social norms and has helped our culture redefine health as merely the absence or presence of symptoms. So even as people feel better when their symptoms are suppressed, they gradually become sicker and sicker, and they never have the chance to address the lifestyle behaviors that are putting them in this potentially fatal situation. It is a vicious cycle.

---

[89]   Diane Vaughan, *The Challenger Launch Decision: Risky Technology, Culture, and Deviance at NASA* (Chicago: University of Chicago Press, 1996).

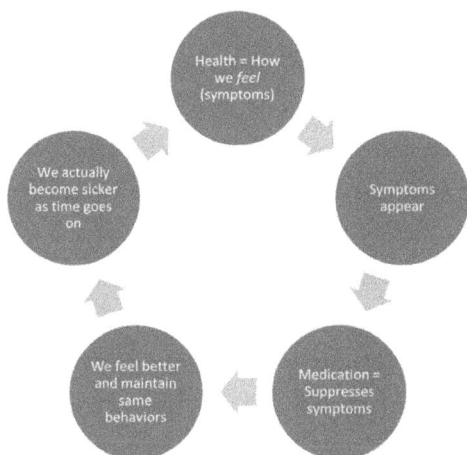

This is the root cause of our health problems. From an outside-in perspective, it is easy to read statistics and headlines and understand that the quality of health in the United States is poor. But that isn't news to anyone these days. Using RCA and looking deeper, we can see extremely concerning practices within politics and medicine that significantly contribute to these poor health statistics. Looking back in history and asking, "Why is this awful behavior so normal and unchallenged," we can clearly see the answer. The past one hundred years of the AMA's efforts have been focused on stamping out holistic perspectives on health, bolstering medical authority, and ensuring that the processes by which science is conducted, health education is taught, and research is paid for come through one single voice. The Flexner Report helped push those first few dominoes.

And now we can see the subconscious effect all of these practices and normalized behaviors have on the American people. Our views on health have been deeply warped. But health is nuanced, subtle, and dynamic. The reason why our modern medical institutions, industries, and corporations continue to fail the American people is that we allow our *beliefs* to be *defined* for us. We allow industries and corporations to redefine what normal is. The number of young children on ADHD medication has almost doubled, pediatric diabetes is exploding, and cardiovascular events are at record highs.[90] We have completely normalized these awful conditions and become numb and desensitized. The system is technically not broken; it is working just as it was designed, to treat and manage *symptoms*. But by only supplying one or two solutions (drugs and surgery), it has created and manipulated what the problem is. It's like the general contractor who shows up at the job site and has only one tool in his bag, a hammer. Everything starts looking like a nail at that point.

To be clear, there are several different kinds of health care providers in this country, and they all serve a critical purpose. To compare the usefulness of a cardiovascular surgeon with that of a nutritionist is not helpful. They both provide essential services, just at varying levels. If you are actively experiencing a cardiac emergency such as congestive heart failure or a gastrointestinal crisis such as appendicitis, you're probably not thinking about holistic solutions and calling up your nutritionist or naturopath. In the event of emergencies, you appropriately seek out emergency care. Most people in the United States do not experience emergencies on a daily or weekly basis; however, their health can still be considered poor. They may experience signs and symptoms frequently, such as shortness of breath, heartburn, apnea, numbness, and tingling, to name

---

[90]   *Cleveland Clinic Journal of Medicine*, "ADHD: Diagnosis and Management in Children and Adolescents," *Cleveland Clinic Journal of Medicine* 84, no. 11 (2017): 873–881, https://www.ccjm.org/content/84/11/873.

a few. Perhaps activities of daily living are becoming increasingly more difficult, such as bathing, getting up and down stairs, and strenuous activities. People in this category more than likely seek out preventive-maintenance health care. They want to ensure that these signs, symptoms, or disabilities do not in any way get worse.

Finally, every year, more and more individuals seek out health care providers that help people promote and optimize their current levels of health. You may experience few to no symptoms in your daily life, but you know that true health is not static. Biological organisms naturally decay and either move in the direction of healing or in the direction of death. You know that your body can always become more resilient. It's why private health practices are exploding across the country. Facilities that specialize in blood chemistry, neurological health, musculoskeletal health, mental health, and so on are being sought out like never before so that individuals can protect and optimize their health and well-being rather than waiting for symptoms to develop.

To undo the damage and social conditioning created by pharmaceutical and medical industries, we must start appropriately designating different kinds of health care providers. Perhaps the first tier of health care should be reserved solely for the emergency treatment of a disease or condition. As we established at the very beginning of this journey, emergency health care professionals (nurses, medical doctors, EMTs) are some of the most overworked and underappreciated professionals in our country. They are victims of our current health care system, with record burnout rates, depression, and anxiety. And more than ever in history, they are departing from their careers. How nice would it be if the only people who used this first tier of health care were the only ones who actually needed these emergency services?

In other words, what if there were a clearly defined second tier? How nice would it be if millions of patients had alternate options for seeking health care before an emergency? Sadly, many people do not have the desire to proactively tend to their health on a daily basis. Whether because of a lack of finances, support, or education, they will settle for simple management of their conditions. Preventing conditions from getting worse is critical if we wish to minimize fatal medical errors and reduce overall mortality rates in our country. This second tier of health care could be the most widely inhabited tier in our country.

The simple distinction between emergency care and preventive health care could make a significant difference in the daily health practices of our country. However, we need a dramatic reformation from the inside out if we wish to see the quality changes we want. The problem with these first two tiers of health care is that they are largely in the hands of pharmaceutical companies and medical institutions that base their work off of symptoms. Until research practices are corrected and finances become more transparent, we cannot place the entirety of our trust or health in those hands. We do need to change the system to see improvements in our collective health. Thomas Edison famously said, "The doctor of the future will give no medicine but will instruct his patient in the care of the human frame, in diet, and in the cause and prevention of disease."

Perhaps the system, as it is, can remain untouched for now. There is one more question worth exploring together. A question we asked at the very beginning of all of this: What do we stand to gain by diverging from this system?

CHAPTER 8

A CROSSROADS

"You cannot change your destination overnight, but you
can change your direction overnight."

—Jim Rohn

I HAVE ALWAYS BELIEVED in the power of choice. Choosing to act based on your own convictions will ultimately be more meaningful than simply doing what you have been told. I also believe we are in a critical time with regard to our individual—and collective—health. It's a fork in the road, if you will. We have the option of continuing down our current path, and by doing so, more than likely we will continue to see the same patterns of results: increases in chronic disease; the continuing decline in the well-being of our children; the collapse of our medical infrastructure; and increasingly adverse conditions for our nurses, medical professionals, and medical students who are in no way equipped (or supported) to keep up with the demand for their services. Down this road, we will continue to see our national debt soar because of staggering medical costs and uneducated and uninterested political leaders arguing for who should be footing the costs of health care while being paid and lobbied by pharmaceutical industries (who win when the people in our country aren't given any other options than what's being sold).

We can continue to believe that the absence of bodily symptoms means that there are no immediate threats to our health and that the average American lifestyle does not need to be changed. We can keep teaching our children about the dangers of bacteria and viruses while overlooking the bodily environments and conditions in which bacteria and viruses thrive. We can keep advertising for the latest drugs that combat X/Y/Z condition and give no attention to the behaviors that enable X/Y/Z to develop.

Or perhaps…we can create the possibility of something *different*—a way of approaching health within a whole new paradigm, a new way of thinking about health, teaching about health, and practicing health. We are talking about a model of health care that is just as applicable to those who live with clearly defined diseases and conditions as it is to those who live free of any symptoms. It's a paradigm of health and well-being that infants and toddlers can participate in alongside senior citizens and everyone in between.

What do *we* stand to gain on a community level when our kids can thrive, more adults can be of contribution rather than of burden, and our medical facilities aren't maxed out?

What do *we* stand to gain on a national level when the quality of life improves, when infant mortality declines, and when academic and public organizations can return to being the natural innovators of health rather than corrupt corporations?

What do *you* stand to gain when you have the power to influence your health and healing on a level for which no one, up until now, has ever given you permission? How would your relationship with your family change? How would it feel to be able to do more of what you love or to spend more time with the people you love? We stand to gain everything if we choose to diverge from what we've been taught and sold.

And it starts with *awareness*: simply being aware of the options that are in front of us. I hope that, at this point on our journey together, it's clear to you that we have been slowly dissecting the mainstream traditional paradigm of health care, how it developed over time, and how it's failing us on a monumental level. The root cause analysis has, for now, been completed. But our work is not yet done. Before rejecting the status quo, we must clearly recognize the alternative health paradigms that exist around us so that you can make an empowered choice for yourself and your family. Being healthy is not an accident, just as our country's health problems aren't an accident. Everything around us can be traced back to deep, systemic causes, both positive and negative. Let's identify the root cause (or causes) of excellent health and vitality, starting with a key distinction: allopathic vs. holistic. With regard to allopathic medicine, it is the traditional or mainstream medical approach that uses drugs, surgery, and other interventions to treat or suppress symptoms and diseases. When you go to a hospital, ER, or outpatient medical clinic, you are more than likely receiving allopathic treatment.

Allopathic medicine, commonly referred to as "Western medicine," is what most of our mainstream health care consists of. On the opposite end of the spectrum is *holistic* health care. Most people today have heard the word *holistic*, but they can't clearly define it, much less understand its role in health care.

Holistic means considering the whole system or person, not just individual parts, with a focus on overall balance and well-being.

Parts versus the whole. Compartmentalized versus an intricately connected system. Both health philosophies are critical. There will always be a necessity for emergency and crisis care, for cutting-edge surgery that saves lives, and skilled diagnosticians to identify and treat life-threatening diseases. Without a doubt, allopathic medicine has been instrumental in the advancement of humanity. But allopathic medicine most certainly needs holistic health care as well, now more than ever. It is a symbiotic relationship. But sometimes it also can remind us of that popular children's toy, the Shape-O Toy Block, with the differently shaped blocks that fit into their corresponding holes. How frustrating it is to watch a child trying to jam triangle-shaped blocks into star-shaped holes.

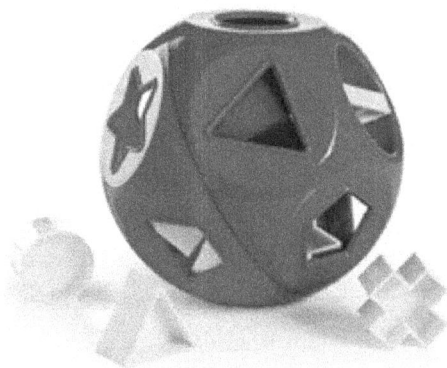

Can we stop forcing millions of Americans to participate in a model of health care that they don't need or desire, or both? Can we capture more Americans who are on the brink of needing emergency crisis care and help them back on the right track into a more preventive model of health? Can we provide such a model to those living among us who not only wish to prevent illnesses but also wish to *promote* health and optimize their own functioning?

Holistic health care provides just that.

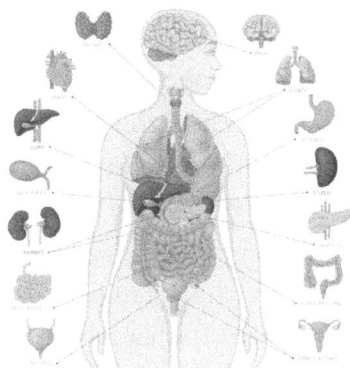

*

Holistic means considering the whole system or person, not just individual parts, with a focus on overall balance and well-being.

Together we will explore what emerges when we shine the spotlight on holistic health care—its practices, its tools, and perhaps most importantly, its *philosophy*. A true holistic provider, whether a doctor of chiropractic, a doctor of osteopathy, a doctor of naturopathy, or even a holistic doctor of medicine, recognizes the indisputable fact that the human body operates as a *whole*. You cannot treat the heart without affecting the kidneys and lungs, and what goes on in the microflora of the gastrointestinal tract affects the biochemistry of the brain. A holistic view of the body understands and accounts for environmental toxins in personal care products that can contribute to the formation of certain cancers. It acknowledges that incorrect rotation of a newborn's cervical spine can cause latching problems and subsequent reflux and other gastrointestinal issues.

Holistic providers teach their patients and their community that the body was designed to be healthy. A simple concept, right? If you were to ask a hundred random strangers, "Was the human body designed to be healthy?" you would probably hear most of those folks say "Of course!" But statistically, we would also expect that sixty-six of those one hundred individuals would be on one form of pharmaceutical medication or another. Many would test positive for having high blood sugar and high blood pressure. A common struggle within the holistic community is reestablishing the difference between "common" and "normal." For holistic fertility and menstrual health providers, it may be *common* to see a community with many young women on estrogen birth control who have irregular periods, excruciating cramping, heavy bleeding, or other menstrual irregularities, but it is certainly not *normal*.

So, what *is* normal for the human body? What is normal health and well-being for all people across the spectrums of age, socioeconomic class, and race? Back to the Shape-O analogy—why do we keep allowing the allopathic model to define *normal* for us? We know what a person's shape is in that model—the person's boundaries begin and end with symptoms. But shouldn't normal be defined by the health experts who specialize in *optimizing* your health?

One of the key distinctions between allopathic health care and holistic health care can be found within their areas of focus. Like allopathic doctors, many holistic providers treat conditions, symptoms, or diseases; however, they do this by using minimal to no medication, modifying lifestyle to the patient's benefit, and treating the body as a whole. As skilled as holistic health care is at understanding and addressing diseases and symptoms, holistic providers differ dramatically from allopathic medicine with their focus on what conditions and factors make a person *healthy*. Not what keeps them from being sick, not what it takes to suppress a symptom, but rather, what contributes to that person's overall well-being and vitality?

These questions were front and center for Aaron Antonovsky and his life's work on *salutogenesis*. Antonovsky was an American Israeli sociologist. After the Second World War, he moved to Israel to begin his epidemiological studies on various ailments. During his work with women going through menopause, he identified those who had survived the concentration camps. To Antonovsky's pure shock, many of these women were able to uphold healthy habits and had high-quality health despite having gone through unspeakable horrors. "How the hell can this be explained?" asked Antonovsky.[91] At that point, he abandoned his work of studying specific diseases and devoted the rest of his life to understanding health and what *causes* it. If this were a root cause analysis of health, salutogenesis would provide the framework for holistic healing to exist.

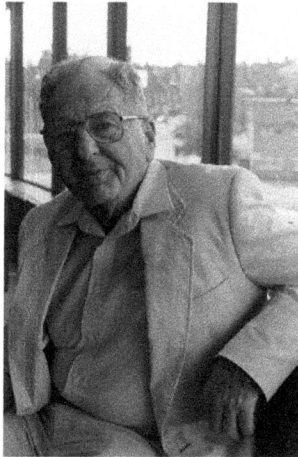

Aaron Antonovsky, the father of Salutogenesis

---

[91] Bengt Lindström and Monica Eriksson, "Contextualizing Salutogenesis and Antonovsky in Public Health Development," *Health Promotion International* 21, no. 3 (September 2006): 238–244.

One of the biggest contributions Antonovsky made to the world of holistic health and healing was the concept of the *health ease/dis-ease continuum.*[92] Within this model, health simply exists as a position on a continuum, rather than health and disease being opposites. The allopathic way of thinking about the human body says, "If you're not healthy, you must be sick and diseased." But health is not binary, not black and white. Antonovsky correctly pointed out that "disease and stress occur everywhere and all the time." However, it is incorrect to assume that stressful experiences are inherently bad or that they *always* cause disease. Under the salutogenic model, stress leads to tension within our bodies; however, the physical outcome (illness, sickness, injury…or healing) is entirely dependent on the adequacy of our *body's ability to manage that tension.*

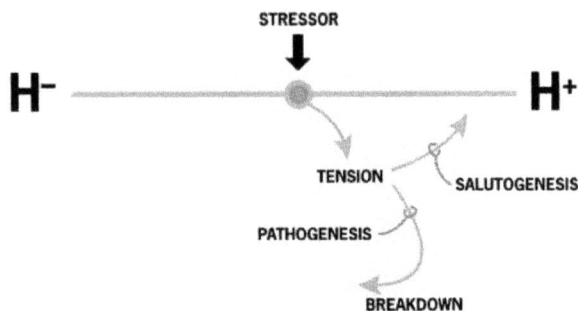

STRESSOR

H⁻ ———————————— H⁺

TENSION   SALUTOGENESIS

PATHOGENESIS

BREAKDOWN

Antonovsky's health continuum illustrates that stress
is not inherently good or bad—what matters is how
the body responds. Depending on one's capacity to
manage tension, the same stressor can lead to breakdown
(pathogenesis) or growth and healing (salutogenesis).

---

[92]   Monica Eriksson, Bengt Lindström, and Jarl A. Lilja, "A Sense of Coherence and Health: Salutogenesis in a Societal Context: Åland, a Special Case?" *Journal of Epidemiology & Community Health* 61, no. 8 (2007): 684–688.

Think of the six strings on a guitar. The strings vary in thickness, and each is tuned to its own unique tension. If you've ever had to painstakingly tune a guitar, you will know that you can only twist that tuning head so many times before... *snap!*—the string breaks. Being able to physically *adapt* to life stressors is critical in the process of healing.

The concept of adaptation is a recurring theme within this salutogenic model, as well as all holistic healing. What are the mechanisms within the human body that allow us to adapt and overcome stressors, whether they be in the form of physical injury, habitual mental or emotional triggers, or even chemical toxicities? How can two people of relatively the same age and apparent state of health be exposed to the same traumas (physical, mental, or chemical) and exhibit two different expressions of health or illness? Antonovsky and his model of health would point to their differing abilities to adapt to those circumstances. He believes that it's the way an individual perceives life and their ability to manage an infinite number of stressors that determines the resulting health outcome. He refers to this ability as a person's *sense of coherence.* And within the salutogenic model, there are three types of coherence that dictate how we stay healthy.[93]

The first type of coherence is *comprehensibility,* meaning: "Can we make sense of our problem?" Think of the average American citizen. Even if that individual has a four-year college degree, making sense of complex health problems that are often nuanced can be extremely difficult. Now factor in the possibility that if this person is sick, diseased, or injured, it's

---

[93]   Aaron Antonovsky, *Unraveling the Mystery of Health: How People Manage Stress and Stay Well* (San Francisco: Jossey-Bass Publishers, 1987).

even more likely that they will not be making choices in a calm, rational state of mind. Think of the poor grandparent alone in the doctor's room, being diagnosed with a condition he or she has never heard of, having to add yet another pharmaceutical drug into the mix, and feeling even more confused. This individual can feel helpless trying to understand the problem, and even more helpless trying to be proactive. Or consider the immigrant parent in the urgent care clinic being discharged with very specific instructions and having to rely on his or her child for interpretation. Health and health care should not have to be a game of telephone, yet it is for millions of people. People need to be able to make sense of their problem, whether it's an existing disease, condition, or a symptom, or the risk factors and behaviors that will inevitably lead to conditions and symptoms. With regard to health comprehension, education is paramount—specifically, education from experts who regularly help people avoid those conditions from developing and know the specific habits and interventions to use. The second aspect of coherence is related to *manageability*. This concept is by far one of the most overlooked aspects of the health of people in our society. It is no secret that life is stressful. From heated political debates to mass shootings, environmental disasters, and economic turmoil—the list goes on and on. Stress is undeniable and seems to be in everlasting supply, which is why we must be able to manage it. We need to know that the stress we are facing daily 1) can be managed with available resources and 2) *must* be managed with available resources. This is where holistic doctors stand to make the difference in our country, on a much larger level.

Aaron Antonovsky knew that in order for someone to have a complete sense of coherence, there had to be a reason why an individual would strive so hard to reclaim his or her health and hold on to it. If salutogenesis is the study of what makes us healthy, we must all have a known reason as to *why* we wish to be healthy and vibrant. What is our connection to this desired state of health? That is why the third and final aspect of coherence is *meaningfulness*. What does it really mean for someone to be able to live a life of effortlessly managing the stressors that surround us all? It is a question we will certainly expand upon—but first the task of understanding this concept of managing stress.

CHAPTER 9

UNDERSTANDING
TRAUMA

"You never know how far reaching something you may think, say, or do today will affect the lives of millions tomorrow."

—B. J. Palmer, developer of chiropractic

TRAUMA HAS OFTEN been defined as any process or event that has occurred too fast, too often, too soon, or not often enough. Think about the traumas that have occurred throughout your life. You may be thinking about that one time you were sitting at a red light when the car behind you smashed into your bumper. *Ouch!* That sudden impact caused incredibly fast hyperextension of your neck, followed by hyperflexion, which placed tremendous amounts of pressure on the facet joints in your cervical spine, (possibly) tearing the microscopic ligaments surrounding them. What about the vape pen that your boyfriend brings with him everywhere he goes? He's happy because he was able to quit smoking and replace it with vaping. But more than likely he doesn't think about the metals and metalloids being propelled into his lungs and bloodstream every time he uses it.

When most people hear the word trauma, they remember incredibly emotional times in their lives—a messy divorce, being fired, the devastating loss of a loved one. Sometimes these emotional traumas keep adding up and their effects become chronic. We don't consciously think about the high levels of cortisol our body secretes in response to these emotional traumas. Or the fact that chronically high cortisol levels attack our bone integrity. Or that they can cause cardiovascular disease. Or that they can even affect the structural integrity of our brain. Within chiropractic philosophy, we find the concept of the *Three T's*: thoughts, traumas, and toxins. The Three T's are what we mean when we use the word *stress*. It can be *physical*, resulting from a car accident. Or *mental*. Or *chemical*. Stress may be classified as a macrotrauma if it's major, such as a car accident or the death of a loved one. Smaller and usually more frequent traumas exist, referred to as microtrauma, and they include such things as continual texting on screens or daily consumption of processed foods.

Living organisms are dynamic, constantly fluctuating. At any given moment we are moving toward repair, regeneration, and healing. Or else we are moving in the direction of decay, illness, injury, or death. It's entirely dependent on how the body adapts to stresses. Whether you're a single-celled organism such as an amoeba or you consist of trillions upon trillions of cells, the body will respond to stressors in one of these two ways. Let's consider the cells for a moment. After all, they are the building blocks of our entire existence. Cellular physiology is a bewildering field of science. For most people, our understanding of cells consists of the last few things we've managed to remember from high school. Terms such as *mitosis, cell membrane,* and *mitochondria* may ring a bell. The important thing to remember is that cells are *always* responding to external stress.

Sometimes the cells respond to trauma by shrinking in size. This is called *atrophy.* Have you ever had to wear a cast for several weeks or even months? Not using your arm muscles for all that time is a trauma for muscle cells that require regular use. When the cast comes off, people can often clearly see smaller, thinner muscles in the injured arm. *Disuse atrophy* of the muscle cells has occurred. There are several other kinds of cell atrophy, some hormonal in cause, some related to nerve damage, and some related to blood-flow issues.

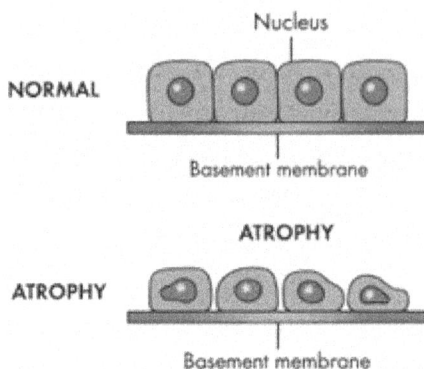

Some types of stress will lead to the enlargement of cell size, otherwise known as *hypertrophy.* Let's stay on the topic of muscle tissue. If increased demand is placed on the muscular system, the muscle tissue will respond by enlarging. Hypertrophy may be completely normal and healthy, like the effects of working out in the gym. It can also be pathological, such as when muscles in and around the heart enlarge.

Normal cell

Increase in
the size
of cells

Hypertrophy

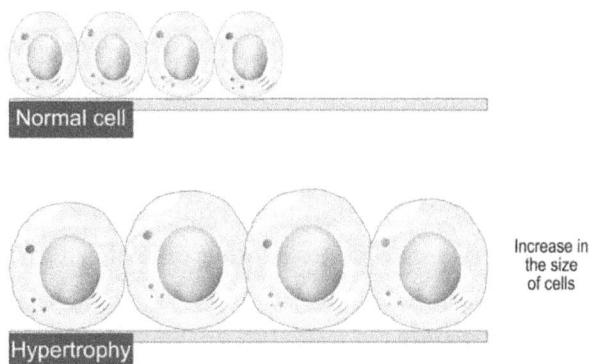

Cellular changes aren't always about cell size. Sometimes the cells within tissue multiply in numbers, leading to an increase in the size of the tissue or organ. This is called *hyperplasia*, and it occurs more commonly than you may think. Hyperplasia occurs in the breast tissue of pregnant women, and it can occur in the hands and feet of physical laborers. Ever had a callus from doing yard work all day? Or consider cigarette smoke. It should go without saying that cigarette smoke is incredibly traumatic to your body, and when we look at the cells within the trachea, we can clearly see how smoke causes cellular injury. In a healthy trachea, the cells are classified as *ciliated columnar epithelial* cells. This means that the cells are shaped like long columns with cilia attached on top that act like little pieces of hair. These cells secrete fluid, help transport material, and act as protective barriers. With chronic exposure to smoke, these cells will eventually be forced to change their shape and overall type in order to survive.

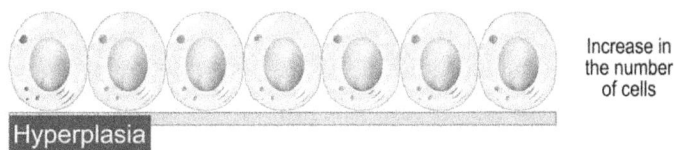

Increase in
the number
of cells

Hyperplasia

Instead of being ciliated columnar cells, they will start to morph into *stratified squamous epithelial* cells. These are flat cells that secrete much less protective fluid, and they are rougher in order to protect against the outside environment. In fact, these cells are commonly found in areas where exposure to the outside environment is more common. The reversible change of one type of cell into another type of cell is referred to as *metaplasia*.

One final example of how cells are always responding to trauma can be illustrated by *dysplastic* change. Sometimes when the cells are constantly being irritated or are chronically inflamed, they can grow in abnormal shapes, sizes, and numbers. This kind of cellular morphology is considered to be *deranged cell growth* and is referred to as dysplasia. A common instigator of dysplasia is the human papilloma virus (HPV). Over time, the cells within the cervix may start to change and appear unrecognizable.

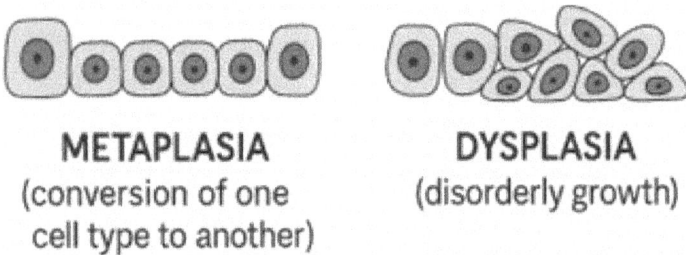

METAPLASIA
(conversion of one
cell type to another)

DYSPLASIA
(disorderly growth)

Regardless of our awareness of the microscopic building blocks that make up our body, the life cycles of cells perfectly illustrate the idea that living organisms are constantly responding to stressors. For instance, *erythrocytes*, or red blood cells (RBCs), are produced within the red bone marrow at a rate of two million cells per second. The process through which RBCs become fully developed and functional is entirely dependent on a few factors. For one, it takes a systemic lack of oxygen in order for the necessary hormones to initiate the process of RBC production. Then, as the immature cell is near formation, it takes adequate supplies of iron, B12, and folic acid for the RBC to be fully developed and functional. Deficiencies in any of these nutrients will lead to a deficiency of RBCs and their reduced functionality or overall oxygenation, otherwise known as anemia.

Trauma of any kind can affect the process of RBC generation. Chronic alcohol use, for example, can lead to lower levels of production as well as abnormally shaped RBCs. Nutritional deficiencies can cause an inadequate supply of B12 or folic acid within the body, again leading to issues with production. After 100–120 days of life, the RBC will eventually undergo the process of programmed cell death. In this process, special cells called *macrophages* physically ingest the old, decaying blood cell, making space for new healthy RBCs that are being produced. The rate at which all these millions of RBCs are killed off and cleared out happens at the same rate new RBCs are being made. This perfect state of equilibrium is critical for the health of all organs in the body, the tissues, and the human body as a whole. What happens to tissue when blood supply is diminished? What happens to our cognitive abilities when less blood is getting to where it needs to? This constant state of RBC production *and* death is essential.

Before its 120 days are up, that RBC desperately needs to survive and remain healthy. The cell is up against significant stress, both physical and chemical. It risks tearing its cell wall when attempting to travel and squeeze through capillaries. We've already pointed to the fact that substances such as alcohol can change the physical shape of the cell, weakening it. Smoking can cause a shrinkage of the actual blood vessel, further narrowing the space that the cell has to travel through. During its lifespan, the RBC, in the face of all these traumas, is either moving in the direction of health and maintenance or quickly toward premature death and decay.

Every single cell, tissue, and organ within the body responds to stress either by repairing and regenerating or by becoming weaker and more dysfunctional, eventually dying. That's what living organisms do; regardless of their physical limitations, they will always attempt to repair. That's why the concept of *adaptation* can apply to a young, vital twenty-year-old the same as to a seventy-five-year-old who has had multiple surgeries and is on multiple medications. Now this seventy-five-year-old may not be healing or regenerating on a cellular level at the same *rate* as the twenty-year-old, but this does not mean that positive physiological actions aren't taking place. We all heal, or break down, at different speeds.

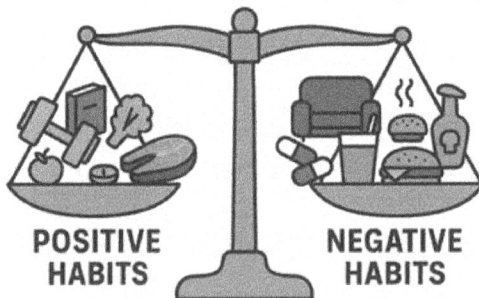

POSITIVE HABITS   NEGATIVE HABITS

Think of a scale. On one end of the scale are all of the healthy, positive habits you have or have had in your life, such as routine physical exercise, disciplined nutritional habits, supplementation, prayer, community, and healthy relationships. On the other end of the scale are all of the traumatic, stressful habits you have had throughout life: sedentary living, vaping or smoking, poor food habits, toxic relationships, and substance abuse. Which side holds more weight? Depending on where your overall health is on any given day, month, or year, you may be able to withstand significant stressors without having any significant breakdown. We've all heard of the word *resilience*, which means "the capacity to recover quickly." How fast can you bounce back? That will be entirely dependent on how your body can *adapt* to the stressors around it on a daily basis.

Each of us has a unique individual threshold for stressors. When we are exposed to more trauma than we can adapt to, well, then we see cells dying, organs becoming dysfunctional, and our bodies becoming sick and diseased. If we want to be able to live within a *holistic* model of health, if we want to break the chains of allopathic thinking and adopt the salutogenic view of health, we need to use the tools and resources around us to effectively adapt to and manage the stressors we are exposed to daily. But what does it mean to "manage"? We've already established that it's not just the suppressing of the symptoms. No, that's not managing anything. What does it actually look like for the human body to manage the trauma that it's been exposed to in life and all the future traumas it's going to be exposed to?

It has to start with how the body communicates.

CHAPTER 10

A WELL-
ADJUSTED LIFE

"Communication with oneself is where all transformation begins."

—Byron Katie

T
O EFFECTIVELY MANAGE any trauma, stressor, or condition within the body, the body must be able to have optimal neurological communication *afferently* (conducting inward) from the cells, the tissues, and the organs up through the spinal cord to the brain, and, at the same time, optimal communication *efferently* (conducting outward) from the brain down through the spinal cord to every aspect of the body it is responsible for healing and repairing.

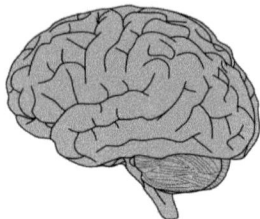

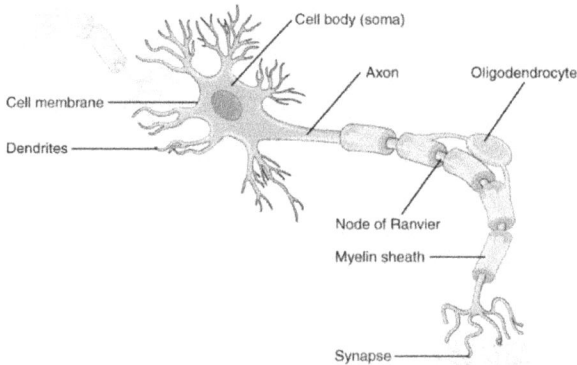

A neuron—the fundamental unit of the nervous system—transmits information through electrical impulses and chemical signals, enabling communication throughout the body.

Within our brain, there are 86 billion cells, called *neurons*. These cells, which vary in shape, size, and function, electrically communicate with each other in networks throughout the entirety of the brain. These neuronal networks allow for executive decision-making; memory formation; the ability to perceive our environment through our senses; the ability to act in the moment; balance; autonomic functions such as heart rate and blood pressure; and more. Pretty much every vital function of our life is the result of these 86 billion neurons doing their job. Now, it is important to note that this critical neurological communication doesn't stay in the brain. This beautifully intricate, amazingly designed system of nerve cells, tissues, and electrical impulses we refer to as the nervous system extends down from the brain through a narrow opening in the bottom of the skull, the *foramen magnum*. At this point, it's a thin, elongated structure called the *brain stem*. Although that name may suggest a division or separation from the brain, it's not separate at all; it's actually a continuation of the brain.

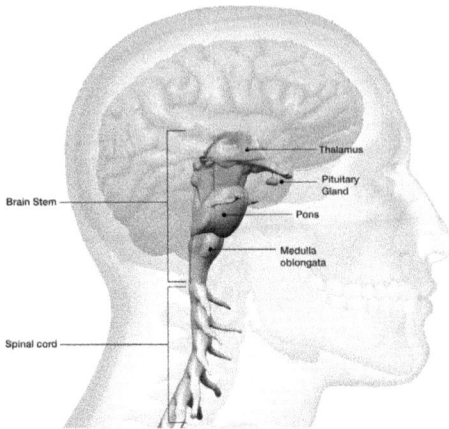

The brainstem exits the skull through the foramen magnum, a large opening at the base of the skull that allows connection between the brain and spinal cord.

Underneath the skull's opening lie the first two *cervical vertebrae* (neck bones). Not only do they allow for mechanical rotation, flexion, and extension of the head but also they provide essential protection to the brain stem as it further transitions into the structure called the *spinal cord*. At this point, our nervous system is no longer confined to the skull; it continues to travel downward housed within the neural canal, the innermost protective column formed by all twenty-four vertebrae of the spine, which are lined up just perfectly to protect and surround the spinal cord all the way down the body. Between each pair of adjacent vertebrae is a small opening called the *intervertebral foramen*. These intervertebral foramina are where the spinal cord branches off into small *nerve roots*. These roots are not separate from the spinal cord, which is not separate from the brain or brain stem.

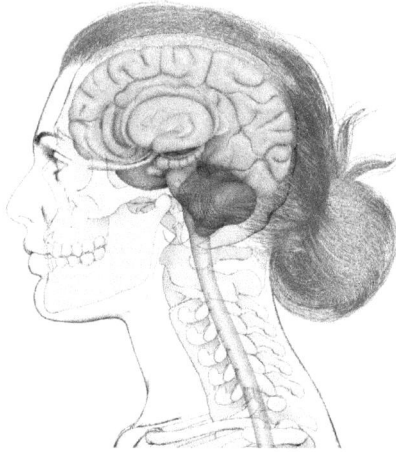

Nerve roots branch off the spinal cord at every level of the
spine, exiting through the intervertebral foramina.

As the cord reaches its maximum eighteen inches, it begins
to branch into thick, fibrous nerve endings called the *cauda
equina*, which then branch off into smaller and smaller nerve
endings shooting down into the legs and lower abdomen. That
is your nervous system, which brings us back to managing *stress*
and *trauma* within the body.

Since 1895, chiropractors have been helping individuals
adapt to the stress in their lives, recover from injuries faster,
and elevate the quality of their health and well-being holistically. All without the use of drugs and surgery. Regardless
of media depiction, chiropractors have been taking care of
children, adults, the sick, the poor, the injured, the uninjured,
and people from practically all walks of life. One reason why
the chiropractic profession is vital in helping shift families
and communities toward a holistic way of living is that it is
one of the only primary care physician groups in America that
acknowledge the fact that *the body is a self-healing organism*. In
fact, the chiropractic profession was built on *that* very premise.

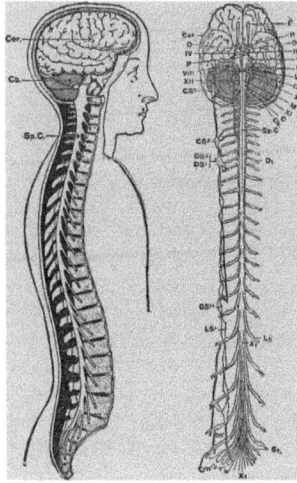

D.D. Palmer introduced the idea of Innate Intelligence—
an inherent guiding force within the body that he believed
coordinated all functions by working through the nervous system.

A hundred years ago, the world's understanding of the human body and its functioning was still fairly limited. However, it was the chiropractic profession that intuitively knew to look within the spine. The chiropractic profession knew that the brain and spinal cord are paramount in expressing vitalism in every function of the body. As science and research around the world and our understanding of neurology advanced, it became clear to chiropractors that the health and functionality of the spine were critical to the normal development of the brain and nervous system. In fact, the acclaimed Nobel Prize–winning neurobiologist Roger Sperry attributes 90 percent of what the brain needs for healthy nutrition, growth, and stimulation to *healthy spinal movement.* So, knowing that the health of the body is dictated by the nervous system's ability to communicate effectively, how does chiropractic fit into that?

Chiropractic most certainly falls under the overarching umbrella of holistic health, as well as the salutogenic model of health. B. J. Palmer, who helped develop the profession into the form we know today, defined chiropractic as "the science, philosophy, and art that utilizes the inherent recuperative power of the body to heal itself. Without drugs or the use of surgery." Simply put: *Chiropractors help people express optimal neurological health by removing specific* interference *to the nervous system.* To accomplish this, doctors of chiropractic assess the spine. All twenty-four vertebrae should have a healthy range of motion, and all the joints within the spine should be properly aligned and have normal joint motion. There are over three hundred articulating joints in the human spine, and they are all surrounded by small encapsulating ligaments that hold those joints delicately together.

Let's leave the spine for now to provide an illustration. Picture your ankle. There is no single bone in the foot called an ankle; rather, the ankle consists of the articulations between the *tibia, fibula, talus,* and *calcaneus* bones. All the bones in each foot are supposed to move in a particular range of motion. When you're jogging down a gravel road and fail to see an uneven spot and roll your ankle, you're forcing all of those tiny joints in directions they don't want to move. Most of the time you're not fracturing these bones when you sprain an ankle. What you are damaging, however, are all of the thick ligaments around your ankle that are responsible for holding these bones in place. Once damaged, these soft tissues can swell and become inflamed and release proinflammatory chemicals into the blood—essentially, all the things that you feel and see when you sprain an ankle.

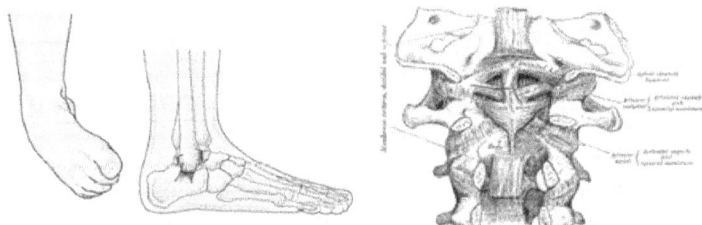

Left: Ankle ligaments. Right: Upper neck spinal ligaments—both stabilize joints and contain mechanoreceptors and proprioceptors that relay crucial movement and position information to the brain.

Now, back to the spine. Together we've established the importance of the spine for your brain's health. Your spine is basically a giant motor for your brain, maintaining neurological health! Unfortunately, it is incredibly common to damage or injure these small spinal joints. We've already described the neural tissue that starts from the brain and ends in your lower back as the spinal cord tapers down. Now let's examine two vertebrae sitting on top of each other.

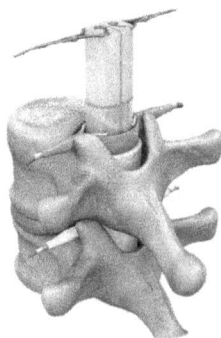

The vast majority of afferent (sensory) input to your brain comes through spinal structures.

Two separate vertebrae are joined together by a large joint called the *intervertebral disc*. The disc is important for many reasons, primarily acting as a shock absorber and creating adequate space for the spinal cord to branch off and form nerve roots that feed into the body. Often overlooked, however, are two additional joints, called *facet joints*. Taken together, these different components are called a *spinal segment*. As with any bony structure in the body (arms, hips, rib cage), muscles and ligaments wrap around these tiny joints in the spine to ensure they maintain proper alignment and to allow for movement.

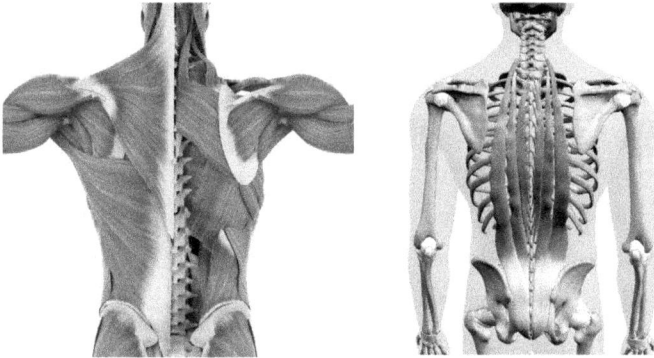

Your spine has both large muscles and small muscles. These smaller muscles contain specialized proprioceptors that provide constant feedback to the brain for spinal alignment and coordination.

These joints, the ligaments around these joints, and all the tiny muscles wrapping up and down the spine are loaded with specialized receptors that send impulses from the spine up to the brain. The brain is constantly listening to these messages. In fact, the brain *depends* on this sensory input from the body to accurately send the right motor commands out. Input in, output out. That's how the body heals, by the way. Being able to accurately understand what's happening, what stress or trauma is being placed on the body, what recovery and repair needs to happen and where—it's all dictated by the brain and, specifically, a few key areas within the brain.

A doctor of chiropractic assesses a person's spine through hands-on analysis and instrumentation to determine which regions of the spine could be causing interference to that person's nervous system. Chiropractors often refer to this interference as *subluxation* or *vertebral subluxation*. This term originated all the way back in the late 1800s to describe the neurological phenomenon observed by Dr. Palmer. Subluxation is a term you may have heard at chiropractors' offices before, and *it is central to the practice of chiropractic.* We've established that all 300+ joints in the spine are innervated with special receptors to enable them to talk to the brain, and that all these joints are surrounded by soft tissue such as ligaments and tiny muscles. We've also established that we need these joints and segments to maintain their healthy ranges of motion. Vertebral subluxation refers to the neurological effects of spinal joint misalignment, the loss of normal joint motion, and the effects of damage to the soft tissue surrounding the spinal segments. Subluxation causes neurological interference in two main ways.

Starting with the spinal segments that are injured, regardless of the type of injury, large or small, when joints are damaged and misaligned, as with the ankle joint, significant swelling and inflammation of the soft tissue around that joint can be triggered. The muscles around the spine can become overactive to try to protect the injury, and over time, the ligaments may become deformed. Remember what exits off the cord between those two vertebrae? Spinal nerve roots. Excessive swelling and inflammation of spinal ligaments and muscles can lead to a buildup of pressure within the spine. All this aberrant pressure easily leads to irritation of the spinal cord or nerve roots. Studies conducted by the University of Colorado show how incredibly sensitive our nervous system is to pressure. The findings indicated: "A pressure of only 10 mm Hg produced a significant conduction block, the potential falling to 60% of its initial value in 15 minutes." That means: the weight of a dime in *pressure* placed on a spinal nerve can reduce its function by up to 60 percent.[94] What is perhaps most concerning about this phenomenon of subluxation (interference) is the fact that it can occur without any perceived symptoms, which is why most people don't think to address this problem until they begin to feel the effects of subluxation weeks, months, or years after an injury.

The second key area in which subluxation causes neurological interference is in the brain itself. Let me introduce to you Dr. Heidi Haavik. Dr. Haavik comes from a family immersed in chiropractic. Her great-grandfather was one of the original students at the Palmer College of Chiropractic, and for Dr. Haavik, it just made sense to become a chiropractor. It was while she was studying for her doctorate that she decided to obtain a PhD in human neurophysiology—the branch of physiology that deals with the functions of the nervous system, initiating her life's work of studying how adjusting the spine truly affects the central nervous system. Dr. Haavik has published numerous papers in chiropractic and neurophysiology journals. She now sits on the editorial boards of the *Journal of Manipulative and Physiological Therapeutics* and the *Journal of Chiropractic Education* and has made monumental contributions to the growing body of evidence for the important conclusion that adjusting subluxated vertebral segments in the spine affects sensorimotor integration in the prefrontal cortex.

---

[94] John Ierano, "Chung-Ha Suh PhD: The Proof of Subluxation. The Final Report of Chiropractic Research at the University of Colorado, 2017," *Asia-Pacific Chiropractic Journal* 2, no. 4 (2021), accessed December 22, 2024.

I've been using a lot of unfamiliar words, so I should quickly define them before we get into the fun world of neuroscience research. Let's start with the brain and its components. Dr. Haavik brilliantly uses the first analogy here. Make a fist, placing your thumb inside. Perfect. Your fingers, thumb, and wrist all represent different aspects of the brain. Your wrist would be your brain stem, critical in unconscious autonomic functions such as heart rate, blood pressure, and breathing. Your thumb signifies your *limbic system*, one of the oldest parts of your brain, and it is highly responsible for controlling your emotions and responding to stress. The four fingers wrapping around your limbic system are your *prefrontal cortex*. The prefrontal cortex, simply put, is how you *reason* and *calm* yourself, an essential function when it comes to managing stress and trauma. When a stressful or traumatic event occurs, your prefrontal cortex is disrupted. Lift your fingers up off your thumb. Without the prefrontal cortex "pumping the brakes" to appropriately inhibit the brain, we begin to operate from our limbic (emotional) system. We become irrational, lose track of time, make emotional decisions, and even perceive our environment differently.

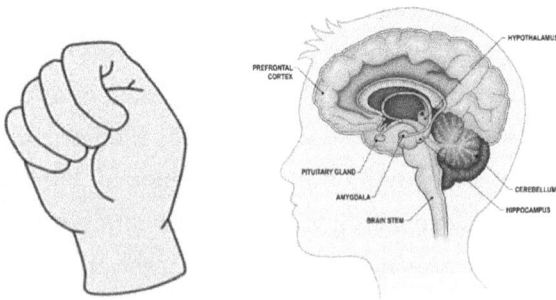

The "Hand Model of the Brain", originally created by Dr. Dan Siegel illustrate how the brain's thinking and emotional parts work together—and what happens when we lose control in stressful moments.

Our prefrontal cortex is responsible for high-level, executive actions within our brain. Functions include:

- Planning a sequence of subtasks to accomplish a goal
- Focusing attention on relevant information and being able to switch attention between tasks
- Inhibiting irrelevant distractors
- Overview of all sensory input
- Monitoring memory
- Response activation and inhibition
- Performance monitoring
- Reward-based learning
- Self-awareness

As Dr. Haavik puts it, our prefrontal cortex is the musical conductor of the brain!

In their article in the *Journal of Neural Plasticity*, Dr. Haavik and her team were able to identify the effect that the chiropractic adjustment has within the brain. Before the chiropractic adjustment, subjects lay on their back while electrical stimulations were given to nerves located in their wrist. During these nerve stimulations, they had sixty-two electrodes on their scalp gathering this signal information. Some subjects received a true chiropractic adjustment, and some received only a sham adjustment that mimicked a genuine chiropractic adjustment.

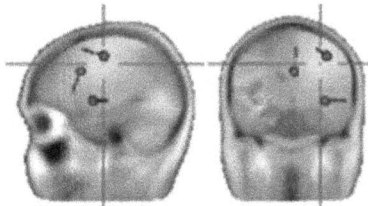

This study shows that spinal adjustments can positively influence how the prefrontal cortex functions, especially in how it processes sensory input and coordinates movement.

The results of this study reproduced findings of earlier studies on chiropractic. Astonishingly, a single chiropractic adjustment of subluxated spinal segments alters how the pre-frontal cortex processes somatosensory information.[95] In more plain language, the chiropractic adjustment improves how the brain takes in information. This published research and other papers since 2016 have laid the groundwork for decades more of legitimate, genuine neuroscientific research into the implications of chiropractic care. Being able to observe changes in the prefrontal cortex, in real time, erases the old mainstream narrative that tried to limit chiropractic to being valuable only for adults with neck or low back pain. The world now has a clear understanding, backed by published research indicating what chiropractors and patients have known for over one hundred years: *Chiropractic is about brain function.*

But not everyone embraces the science. Take Australia, for instance. In 2019, Victoria health officials issued a survey across the state asking parents about their experiences (if any) in bringing their children to a chiropractor. The reality of the situation was that the Australian government was attempting to suppress children's access to chiropractic care. Concerns about safety and efficacy, stemming from bias and ignorance, led to the distribution of thousands of surveys across the state to gather information trying to confirm the beliefs of their already made-up minds.

---

[95] Heidi Haavik et al., "Manipulation of Dysfunctional Spinal Joints Affects Sensorimotor Integration in the Prefrontal Cortex: A Brain Source Localization Study," *Neural Plasticity* 2016 (2016): Article ID 3704964.

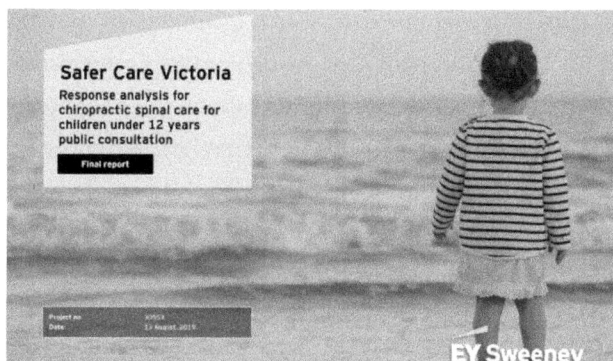

What the officials were not expecting to get in return was overwhelming public support for pediatric chiropractic care. Over twenty-one thousand surveys were filled out, answering a variety of health-related questions. Within the past 10 years, 21,824 people have responded saying that they received chiropractic care along with their children. The average age of a child brought to a chiropractor was 2, and 99.7 percent of the respondents were supportive of chiropractic care for children.[96]

The reasons *why* their children were brought to chiropractors varied. Postural concerns topped the list (31.7 percent), with colic coming in at a close second (28.7 percent). Other answers were breastfeeding issues, headaches, walking problems, crawling, and bedwetting. In addition, a significant number of responses were "other," and when those parents were further questioned, they referenced "general health and well-being / preventive care / alignment" as the primary reason they sought chiropractic care for their children.

How satisfied were the twenty-one thousand parents with the information they received from their chiropractor about the benefits of care? Responses indicate that 99.1 percent were

---

[96]   *Safer Care Victoria, Chiropractic Spinal Manipulation of Children Under 12: Independent Review*, October 2019, accessed December 22, 2024.

either *satisfied* or *very satisfied*. When it came to the satisfaction rating for education provided by other/alternative providers, such as medical providers, ratings dropped to 78.9 percent. As to the actual results and health benefits these parents noticed, 98.3 percent of them indicated that the child receiving chiropractic care was either *somewhat improved* or *much improved*.

Now, twenty thousand positive survey responses may not carry the same weight as a randomized clinical control trial, but this does not negate the significance of a government-sponsored health survey. Over twenty thousand parents sought out chiropractic care for their young children and were more than happy and pleased with their experiences, both clinically and personally. One parent noted, "As they grow, I consider regular chiropractic checks to be part of our family health regime, just like regular medical and dental checks, I consider it setting a strong foundation for their future health." In a world where Western allopathic medicine is the primary form of health care, this survey is a humbling reminder that we have no shortage of holistic tools at our disposal. We just have to know where to look. Here is what one anonymous parent said: "It has been a remarkable recovery and of great interest to all of the doctors involved in my son's care. He was recently discharged by the pediatric gastroenterologist. The ENT surgeon said that surgery wasn't necessary, and the doctors remained perplexed by my son's radical recovery of his health problems from chiropractic treatments." [97]

See what's possible when we treat the body as a whole rather than just parts? At this point, if you are unfamiliar with chiropractic care, the neurology around it, and its applicability

[97]   *Safer Care Victoria, Chiropractic Spinal Manipulation of Children Under 12: Independent Review*, October 2019, accessed December 22, 2024.

to both adults and children, you might be wondering about the results of chiropractic care in the United States. What is the benefit to patients under chiropractic care? We know it's holistic in its philosophy. We know it's natural. But what kind of results are people actually receiving?

Dr. Richard Sarnat is the chief medical officer and president of Advanced Medicine Integration group (AMI). For over ten years, Dr. Sarnat compiled research from one of the nation's largest insurance underwriters studying the effect that chiropractic care has on patients within the medical model of health care. From 1999 to 2002, AMI contracted with chiropractors to serve as primary care physicians (PCPs) within the integrative medicine independent physical association (IPA). The IPA data was published in the *Journal of Manipulative and Physiological Therapeutics* in 2004 and then updated three years later. Clinical and cost utilization based on 70,274 member-months over a seven-year period was compared with conventional medical IPA values. After all of the data were compiled, it was found that the holistic-oriented PCPs *using a nonsurgical/ nonpharmaceutical approach* demonstrated reductions in both clinical and cost utilization when compared with PCPs using conventional medicine alone.[98] Chiropractic patients who were under routine care, when compared with patients who were not under chiropractic care, saw a…

- 60 percent decrease of in-hospital admissions
- 59 percent decrease in hospital days

---

[98]   Richard L. Sarnat, James Winterstein, and Jerrilyn A. Cambron, "Clinical Utilization and Cost Outcomes from an Integrative Medicine Independent Physician Association: An Additional 3-Year Update," *Journal of Manipulative and Physiological Therapeutics* 30, no. 4 (2007): 263–269.

- 62 percent decrease in outpatient surgeries and procedures
- 85 percent decrease in pharmaceutical costs.

The beautiful thing about chiropractic care is that it is not about the treatment of symptoms and conditions. It is about *optimizing* our *nervous system* and its ability to function *better*. It's about restoring normal motion to the spine by adjusting subluxated segments, *allowing our brain to better perceive our own body* so that we can adapt to the stress and trauma we incur in our lives, whether we are asymptomatic children or adults living with frustrating and exasperating symptoms. Chiropractic care can be applied to any part of the health spectrum, whether it is with the intention of maintaining and preserving our health or recovering from injury and illness. Our society tends to think that the simple act of consciously choosing holistic health care over mainstream allopathic health care is an act of *rejecting* mainstream medicine. This isn't really accurate. One Australian parent put it like this: "We should not be dictated to about whether we use natural and preventative care for our own families. Chiropractic care is safer than medical care—the research proves this. This is not to say I don't or wouldn't use mainstream medicine because I do when I have to. I believe an integrated approach where we can use the most appropriate care in the most appropriate situation benefits everyone."

Every single human on Earth should know how to manage the physical, mental, and chemical stress their body is exposed to on a daily basis. We now know that this management of stress really comes down to a cellular level. Where we should start is ensuring—what is innately guaranteed in a *healthy* body—that every single cell, tissue, and organ has the ability to:

- Process information.
- Receive commands.
- Communicate vital information to the central nervous system and receive vital information from it.

If you are attempting to treat and manage symptoms, start with the body's communication pathway. If you are asymptomatic and attempting to optimize your body's health potential, you need to maintain and protect your body's communication pathway.

Chiropractic care does just that.

However, a healthy tree does not have just one singular root; it has multiple roots. By studying the nervous system, it is easy to appreciate the electrical components that make up neurons and the brain and spinal cord. But the human body is also highly chemical in its constituents. Let's now turn our attention to the chemical building blocks that our nervous system depends on for adequate and sufficient use. Yes, we are going to discuss nutrition.

CHAPTER 11

CELLULAR NUTRITION

"Good food is very often, even most often, simple food."

—Anthony Bourdain

N*UTRITION.* E*VERYONE HAS* a unique reaction when they hear that word. Some picture meal prepping, or the condition of their physique, or the various diets they've tried throughout the years. Others immediately feel judged and inadequate, assailed by thoughts of all the nutritional things they think they're not doing right. I assure you, however, that this chapter is not a critique of any individual's nutritional lifestyle or a deep dive into the various diets. It's impossible to have a conversation about nutrition without acknowledging the roles that culture, religion, and social and economic standing play in how we view nutrition. We could easily write an entire book on nutrition (in fact, there are thousands) and the role it plays in our health. So let's remind ourselves what we are talking about right now—holistic healing, and reclaiming our health, and breaking the chains that modern Western allopathic medicine has put around our health journeys. We started our exploration of holistic healing by discussing Aaron Antonovsky and his concept of salutogenesis, i.e., what makes a person healthy. What are the practices; what are the characteristics?

The first is comprehensibility. Can we make actual sense of what is going on with our health? Do we understand the physiological processes going on inside our body? Once we comprehend our health (or illness), we can efficiently manage it. When it comes to managing the stress in our lives, we should always start with our body's *communication pathway*. Ensuring proper neurological development through healthy spinal function is a critical piece in allowing our body to adapt to stress and overcome it, and it's for that reason that chiropractic care is so vital in helping our society heal. However, our nervous system can only do so much. There is a limitation to what can be controlled and regulated within our internal environment, and that comes down to the chemical building blocks with which the body is built. *That* is nutrition.

The very word *nutrition* comes from the Latin word *nutrire*, meaning "to nourish." Today we understand nutrition to be the process by which organisms obtain nutrients, metabolize those nutrients, and use them to support life. Within the United States, entire divisions of academia, research, and government are devoted to the topic of nutrition and how to best study, teach, and address it. As with any health topic, nutrition is particularly sensitive for most people. When we talk about the foods we eat and the nutritional practices we uphold, we're also bringing to the table our heritage, our traditions, our cultures—treasured practices handed down to us.

But also at the table are our food addictions, emotional resentments tied to foods, preconceived notions, and fears of being judged. Discussing nutrition is difficult. And for the sake of the current conversation, let's acknowledge the nuances of nutrition, the breadth of nutritional history, and the beautiful roles that our religions and ethnic backgrounds play in it. And let's acknowledge the racial disparities that exist within the world of nutrition, socioeconomic crisis factors, and the systemic failures in the United States regarding the nutritional education of the public. Finally, let's have a look at the almighty Food Guide Pyramid, a product of the United States Department of Agriculture.

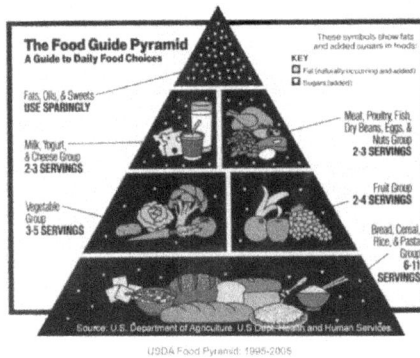

Throughout this discussion we have been analyzing the deep, often hidden roots of our current state of health. At the deepest levels of ourselves, it all comes down to what we *believe* to be true, and this government-curated guideline has been instrumental in forming the basis of what millions of Americans believe to be nutritionally healthy and safe. But before we discover the spectacular ways people can use food and nutrition to gain power over their health, we must first call a spade a spade. The Food Guide Pyramid has done immeasurable harm to our children and our country. Let's understand why. The base of the pyramid alone should be enough to raise red flags. The USDA was aware of the state of the country's health, and it saw chronic illnesses such as coronary artery disease and obesity on the rise, yet it made the bold recommendation of six to eleven servings per day of carbohydrates like bread, rice, crackers, and cereal. As to fats, at a time when the country's concern for heart disease was growing, it might have made sense to limit fatty foods. Unfortunately, the USDA's comprehension of cholesterol and fat was incredibly misguided. They also limited *healthy* fats and substituted dangerous amounts of carbs in their place.

Carbohydrates can be either simple (refined) or complex (natural, found in fruits, vegetables, legumes, and whole grains). Simple, refined carbs are sugars or starches that have been processed and stripped of their natural fiber and other nutrients, such as vitamins and minerals. Refined carbs increase blood sugar levels far more than whole-grain foods do. Now of course there is nothing wrong with keeping blood sugar elevated throughout the day; it's an easy, fast way to give the body energy. But consider the average American student. A typical day for a middle schooler consists of six hours of sitting down—on the bus ride to school, in the classroom, at lunch (no more recess!), and the bus ride home. Those six hours don't even count at-home studying and sitting-down recreational viewing. So we now have a physically underactive child, largely sedentary in lifestyle, whose parents follow the recommendation that they consume six to eleven servings of cereal, pasta, white rice, white breads, and crackers each day. A carb-rich meal will cause the pancreas to respond to this elevated blood sugar by releasing the hormone *insulin* to guide glucose into the bloodstream and then into the muscles and liver. Thank God for the pancreas and insulin (when they are working properly!). But the sugar isn't just from the carbs in our daily meals. A significant problem is that many of us also consume beverages all day long that are loaded with sugar. Consider a seasonal drink found in certain Pacific Northwest–based coffeehouses. One grande Pumpkin Spice Latte in this establishment contains 50 grams of sugar! Add to that a chocolate croissant, and you are well on your way to *insulin resistance.*

Insulin resistance refers to the condition in the body that can occur when a person's diet includes excessive refined carbs, added sugars, and saturated trans fats. As insulin resistance builds, the body no longer absorbs glucose (blood sugar) into the muscles, liver, or fat cells. The sugar in your blood now accumulates, leading to a whole host of health problems: diabetes, fatty liver disease, and cardiovascular diseases. The fact that neither the 1992 nor the updated 2005 Food Guide Pyramids made clear distinctions between refined carbohydrates and whole-grain complex carbs is horrendous, to say the least. Everyone needs to know that not all carbohydrates are good for us.

Unfortunately, that's not the only concept the USDA got wrong. It also failed to educate us on the critical difference between good fats and bad fats. The conversation around different kinds of fat is usually just in the context of cholesterol. To make things clear, we are going to quickly illustrate good and bad fats as well as good and bad cholesterols.

One theory as to the reason the USDA relegated foods such as chicken, turkey, fish, and nuts to the upper, smaller sections of the pyramid was the growing concern over the relation of fat to heart disease—specifically, *cholesterol* and heart disease. What makes this dietary decision all the more frustrating was that researchers have known for years that some kinds of fat and cholesterol are actually essential to human health, and they *protect* the heart. For decades, our country has demonized fats

(*any* fats) in an effort to protect heart health (or perhaps to protect the statin industry), yet here we are in 2025 with 650,000
cardiovascular fatalities a year. Something isn't adding up.

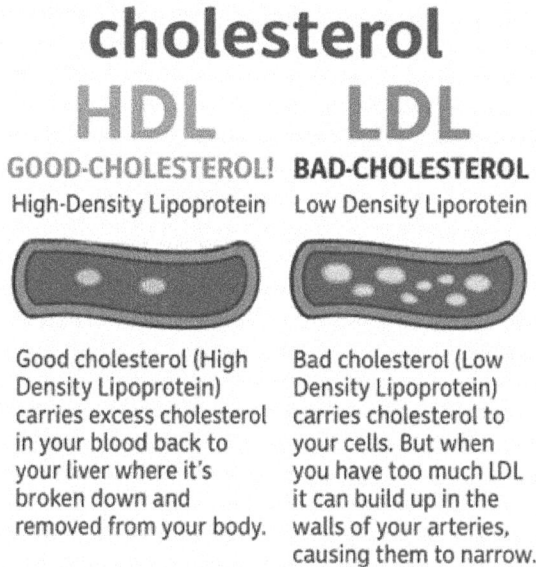

cholesterol
HDL   LDL
GOOD-CHOLESTEROL! **BAD-CHOLESTEROL**
High-Density Lipoprotein   Low Density Liporotein

Good cholesterol (High
Density Lipoprotein)
carries excess cholesterol
in your blood back to
your liver where it's
broken down and
removed from your body.

Bad cholesterol (Low
Density Lipoprotein)
carries cholesterol to
your cells. But when
you have too much LDL
it can build up in the
walls of your arteries,
causing them to narrow.

*

We desperately need healthy fats in our diet. Poly- and
monounsaturated fats that are found in foods such as olive oil,
walnuts, avocados, walnuts, and fish oil help the body raise
high-density lipoprotein (HDL) cholesterol—that is, good cholesterol—and lower the levels of low-density lipoprotein (LDL)
cholesterol, bad cholesterol. HDL takes cholesterol and guides
it back to the liver, thus lowering the amount of cholesterol
found in the bloodstream. LDL, on the other hand, transports
cholesterol molecules throughout the body and contributes to
the buildup of plaque in blood vessels and eventual cardiovascular disease.

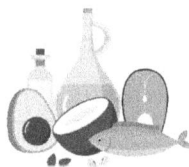

Unsaturated fats   Saturated fats   Trans fats

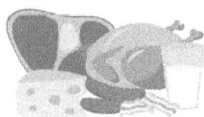

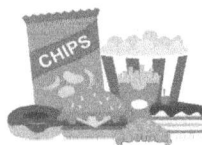

Not all fats are created equal—unsaturated fats (like those in avocados and fish) support heart health, while excess saturated fats and trans fats (often in processed foods) may raise health risks.

And there's more to know about fats. A critical kind of fat that the body is unable to produce on its own is omega-3 fatty acid. This fatty acid is essential to cellular membranes, cellular receptors, and the regulation of inflammation in the body, and it is the precursor to many hormones. Omega-3 is a type of polyunsaturated fat and can be found in walnuts, flax seeds, and fish. What about the other fats out there? Most fat-containing foods have mixtures of fat (unsaturated, saturated, or even trans fats). Foods such as chicken, nuts, or fish contain both kinds of fats, although leaner meats tend to have higher amounts of unsaturated fat. Foods such as ice cream, marbled beef, and cheeseburgers have much more saturated fat. Even certain plant foods, such as coconut oil, palm oil, and palm kernel oil, are rich in saturated fats. Now, it may be easy to view ice cream and cheeseburgers as unhealthy because they are loaded with preservatives, refined carbs, and added sugars, but isn't the saturated fat the main reason? Researchers from the Oakland Research Institute published an extensive meta-analysis studying the association between saturated fats in our diet and cardiovascular disease, coronary heart disease, and stroke. Data were used from twenty-one different studies that followed 350,000 people for up to twenty-three years. Their conclusion, which was published in *The American Journal of Clinical Nutrition*, was, "There is insufficient evidence from prospective epidemiologic studies to conclude that dietary saturated fat is associated with an increased risk of CHD, stroke, or CVD.[99] Wait, what?!

If you are starting to question every piece of nutritional advice you ever heard growing up, you're not alone! Our understanding of nutrition and health has been aggressively manipulated to the point that most people just follow what they were told as a child. As we established at the beginning of this section, nutrition is tricky. It's complicated, and unfortunately, our leading health educators and elected health officials seem to have abandoned their efforts to teach us the subtleties that exist within the world of nutrition. "All fat is bad fat" is much easier to advertise and create infographs around. Even the most extensive study in the world on this matter has been ignored. Sponsored by the Women's Health Initiative, it studied nearly fifty thousand women who were randomly assigned to either a low-fat diet or their usual diet. Those assigned to the low-fat group did *not* significantly reduce their incidence of breast cancer, heart disease, or stroke.[100]

When the USDA decided to wage an all-out war on fat, they created a fatal power vacuum. Fat was out (including the

---

[99]   Patty W. Siri-Tarino et al., "Meta-Analysis of Prospective Cohort Studies Evaluating the Association of Saturated Fat with Cardiovascular Disease," *The American Journal of Clinical Nutrition* 91, no. 3 (March 2010): 535–546.

[100]   Ross L. Prentice et al., "Low-Fat Dietary Pattern and Risk of Invasive Breast Cancer: The Women's Health Initiative Randomized Controlled Dietary Modification Trial," *JAMA* 295, no. 6 (2006): 629–642.

healthy, protective fat) and grains were now in. Low-fat cookies, cereals, chips, and other grains were now being heavily marketed to children. By taking fat out of the diet, of course LDL cholesterol can fall, but so do HDL levels. Low HDL levels *increase* one's risk of heart disease.[101] Again, researchers knew this information before the release of the Food Guide Pyramid.

As the good fats became more and more restricted in the diet, dangerous fats rose. Trans-fatty acids, or trans fats, are made by heating liquid vegetable oils in the presence of hydrogen gas and a catalyst, a process called *hydrogenation*. Trace amounts of trans fat naturally occur in some foods (beef and dairy fat); however, the majority of trans fats are found in hydrogenated vegetable oils (think fried foods, baked goods, processed foods).[102] There are *bad* fats, and this is the worst kind of fat you can put into your body. Trans fats simultaneously raise LDL levels and lower HDL levels. They create inflammation and contribute to insulin resistance. Trans fats are most typically found in (but not limited to) frozen pizza, margarine, store-bought dough, commercially baked goods, microwave popcorn, and fried foods of any kind (because of the chemical transformations from high heat).

Any nutritionist worth his or her salt (no pun intended) can take one glance at the Food Guide Pyramid and see glaring issues. What isn't as obvious is the fact that it was never intended to turn out this way. Perhaps we should hear from the woman who was *supposed* to be responsible for the almost $1 million dollar graphic. Luise Light is considered by many to be an expert on nutrition. She helped develop the National Cancer

---

[101]   Centers for Disease Control and Prevention (CDC), "LDL and HDL Cholesterol and Triglycerides," last modified May 17, 2021.

[102]   *American Heart Association*, "Trans Fat," accessed December 22, 2024.

Institute's first diet and created other nutritional guidelines for cancer patients. She has done extensive work with supermarkets around the country that led to the National Nutrition Labeling Program. And she has served as the USDA Director of Dietary Guidance and Nutrition Education Research. Luise Light dedicated years of her life to help create a healthier and safer generation of children and was responsible for the iconic Food Guide Pyramid we all grew up with. The sad part is that almost none of the research and effort she put into the pyramid project was published.[103]

When Light was first sought out to take on this task, she jumped on the opportunity, writing, "Food guides are a way of translating dietary recommendations for nutrients into food choices. They are the most frequently used devices for teaching about nutrition, and they have a long and proud history." Drawing on her impressive background in public health, she knew the weight of this new project of hers. She knew that offering advice about eating that *didn't* reflect prevention of the major health problems linked to diet would be dangerous and misleading. In her 2006 book, *What to Eat: The Ten Things You Really Need to Know to Eat Well and Be Healthy*, Light shares her memories of her time in Washington, DC, and the uphill battle she fought to bring nutritional awareness to our country's children. Here's a particularly interesting excerpt: "Before my first day on the job, I was invited to dinner with people from the food industry who said they wanted to welcome me to Washington. Naive about the way business is done in the Capital, and curious to know how these food industry executives knew I existed, I accepted the invitation."

---

[103] Luise Light, *What to Eat: The Ten Things You Really Need to Know to Eat Well and Be Healthy* (New York: McGraw-Hill, 2006).

Light went on to say: "They introduced themselves and, as I recall, said they were with the Cattlemen's Association, the Grocery Manufacturers, the National Food Processors, the Meat Institute, the Dairy Council, and the Egg Board. They questioned me about my nutritional opinions: how I felt about the value of butter, eggs, meat, and cholesterol in the diet, what I thought of leading consumer advocates (whom they named), suggesting offhandedly that most of them were either socialists, gay, or anarchists and therefore not to be trusted.

"I doubted this and wondered why they felt the need to discredit them with me."

After this dinner, Light ended up spending several months creating a plan for this new state-of-the-art dietary guide. She ensured that this guide was based on research on current health challenges linked to diet and nutrition patterns and the latest research from the National Academy of Sciences. She even went as far as using computer simulations to create models of what typical meals and snacks should look like based on known public eating patterns. Light put significant effort into ensuring that these new guidelines would have "little or no significant negative economic impact on consumers or the food industry in terms of food expenditures."

Light and her team left no stone unturned in their attempt to create the most evidence-based, practical nutritional and dietary guide. They submitted their final version of the Food Guide Pyramid to the secretary of agriculture. Here is more from her book: "Then something bizarre happened. When the new food guide came back from review by the office of the Secretary of Agriculture, changes had been made to it. The number of servings in the whole grains category had been altered from the original two to three to six to eleven, and the words 'whole grains' were nowhere to be found. Dairy was now three to four servings, protein foods had become two to three servings, and fats, oils, and sweets to 'use moderately,' without further explanation."

The USDA had censored Luise Light and her team's research, auctioning off the Food Guide Pyramid to the highest bidders.

We have a unique opportunity available to us in this present moment. Faced with record-high rates of heart disease, pediatric diabetes, autoimmunity, and cancer, we can help an entire generation of children (and their parents) unlearn the damage done by this standardized dietary "guide" and reclaim their health through nutrition. By now, we know we cannot wait for the government's intervention. Light reminds us: "Ultimately, the food industry dictates the government's food advice, shaping the nutrition agenda delivered to the public. In fact, to the food industry, the purpose of food guides is to persuade consumers that *all* foods (especially those that *they're* selling) fit into a healthful diet."

In the spirit of creating deep roots of health and well-being, let's start by teaching children that the way they approach food and nutrition can set them up to not just overcome sickness, injury, or stress but also to completely shift the way in which they live their lives. Spending extended periods of time with young children can give anyone a pathological resentment toward certain words. *Mine*, if screamed at a specific volume and octave, can send shivers down any parent's spine, even a seasoned one. *No*, when used a certain number of times, can effectively shake an adult's soul. *Why*, however, is a critical question that children use to make sense of their world. This single word is the basis of *root cause analysis* and the catalyst for this entire journey we're on together. Let's help answer our children's questions about *why* they should (or should not) eat certain foods.

We have already established that in order to holistically heal and thrive, we must know how to manage our lifestyle, which includes the stressors we all encounter. Children are not exempt from stressors of any kind. Many health professionals argue that children born today live under more physical, emotional, and chemical stress than did their parents and grandparents. The foods we eat and the drinks we consume directly contribute to our body's resilience against trauma—or they directly set us up to become susceptible to illness and disease. And it starts in the cells. So, back to the biology classroom we go.

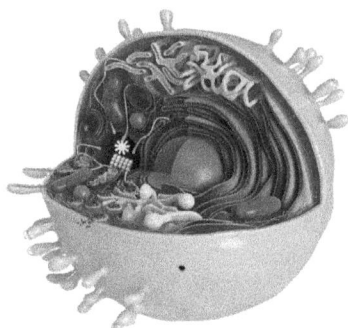

What we are looking at is a human cell. Intricately and beautifully designed, the human body consists of about 37 trillion of these. When similar-acting cells group together to function, they are called *tissue*. Although only tissues and organs are visible to us, this does not mean that cells are inconsequential and have significance only when they come together in a group. Every single cell in your body performs complex functions and even contains smaller structures within itself called *organelles* to deliver energy, strength, and protection to the entire cell.

This diagram simplifies the structure of the cell and makes it easy to identify the various organelles. There are three aspects of the cell that we are going to focus on when it comes to our nutritional journey: the *cell membrane*, the *mitochondria*, and the *nucleus*.

Around each and every one of your cells is a thin, flexible barrier that protects its contents from the outside environment. Sometimes referred to as the *plasma membrane*, but more commonly called the cell membrane, this layer of protection is vital to the survival of your cells. This membrane keeps all the necessary components of the cell, including its nutrients, safe and in one spot, while keeping harmful molecules such as toxins out. In addition to protection, the cell membrane is also vital to transportation along the cell, cell signaling, and cellular recognition. When you look at the actual chemical composition of a cell membrane under a microscope, you can clearly see something called a *phospholipid bilayer*.

That was a mouthful of syllables. What does this mean to you and your health? Simply put, *healthy fats constitute the boundaries of your cells!* And it is this chemical structure that turns your cell membranes into semipermeable filters that allow nutrients to enter and waste to leave. It also allows your cells to communicate with each other, enabling your entire body to achieve *homeostasis* (equilibrium with the environment). Fats, proteins, and some carbohydrates can be found within your cells and most certainly in the cellular membranes. For our cells, what we eat can become either protection and nutrition or harm and destruction.

Let's look at diets high in saturated fats, specifically trans fats. In order to function correctly, our cell membranes are supposed to be flexible, but when we consume foods high in trans fats, our cellular membranes lose their flexible nature and become brittle and rigid, completely impairing the function of the membrane itself.

Consuming healthy fats is essential.

When it comes to protecting your cellular membranes through-out your body, unsaturated fats have been widely known as an important staple of the body's chemical needs.

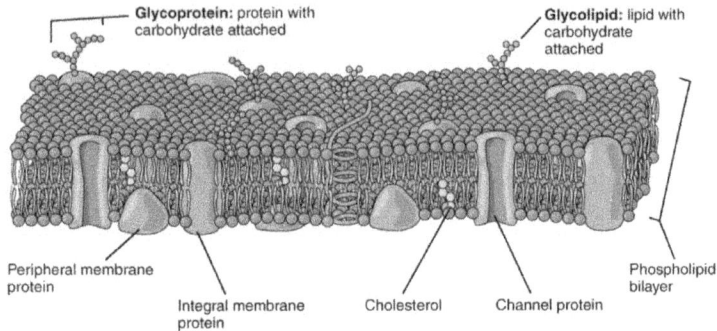

Glycoprotein: protein with carbohydrate attached

Glycolipid: lipid with carbohydrate attached

Peripheral membrane protein

Integral membrane protein

Cholesterol

Channel protein

Phospholipid bilayer

The phospholipid bilayer is the flexible barrier that protects your cells, but its function depends on the fats you eat—healthy fats like omega-3s keep it fluid and responsive, while trans fats make it stiff and dysfunctional.

However, it is important to distinguish between *omega-3* and *omega-6* fatty acids, two categories of unsaturated fats. Foods such as walnuts, almonds, and various types of vegetable oils (sunflower, safflower, canola, peanut) are all rich sources of omega-6 fatty acids. The problem is that these particular fatty acids are terribly proinflammatory. The more omega-6 found in the body, the higher its systemic inflammation tends to be. Because of America's adoration of processed, baked, and fried foods (all using copious amounts of trans fats, vegetable oils, and omega-6), we are a highly inflamed population (not just politically!).

On the other hand, fatty fish (salmon, tuna, cod), hemp seeds, kidney beans, seaweed, flaxseed, and wheat germ are all excellent sources of omega-3 fatty acids. Deficiencies of this

specific fatty acid have been linked to mental health conditions such as depression, anxiety, ADHD, and Alzheimer's
disease. Aside from good quality fats, choline is also an essential cell nutrient, critical during fetal development for the
brain's growth. Choline also plays a central role in the structural
integrity of cellular membranes as well as cell signaling. Choline is easily found in egg yolks and organ meats. Aside from
meat, legumes and wheat germ are good sources of choline.
In summary, a healthy cellular membrane is essential in the
protection of cells, as well as in many other roles. There are,
however, compartments on the inside of the cell that have an
even larger role to play.

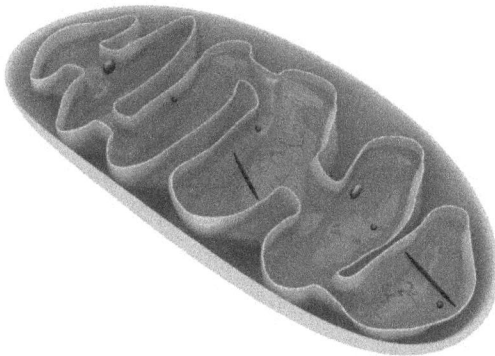

Mitochondria are the cell's powerhouses, and when they're
not functioning properly, energy drops, inflammation
rises, and the risk for chronic diseases like diabetes,
heart disease, and neurodegeneration increases.

If you've ever been tasked with trying to feed a small child
healthy food, you may have used the phrase "food is fuel." But
how does this process really happen, in which our body takes
in food, digests it, and somehow gets it to the microscopic cells
all over our body? This is where the *mitochondria* become of
utmost importance. Mitochondria are found inside the cells of

all animals, plants, and even fungi and are the primary source of energy within the body. They take large molecules from our food (such as carbs or fats) and break them down into usable molecular forms of energy called *adenosine triphosphate* (ATP). Hence the mitochondria's iconic nickname, the "powerhouse of the cell." Without a doubt, mitochondria are essential elements for human survival. Sometimes people are born with mitochondrial disorders, leading to awful problems with their vital organs, especially their muscles, heart, eyes, and nervous system. Mitochondrial disorders can even cause different kinds of cancer.

The conversion of different molecules obtained from our food into actual energy used by the cells is a highly chemical process facilitated by various vitamins and minerals, including a well-known family of eight essential water-soluble vitamins, the B group. Largely because of this water solubility, the body does not store excess amounts of B vitamins, and this requires our diets to be a rich source of this vitamin group. Let's look at the first of these B vitamins, *thiamine* (B1). Ninety percent of cellular thiamine is found within the mitochondria, and it is heavily involved in basic cell functions, including the breaking down of nutrients for energy use. Excellent sources of thiamine include pork, fish, beans, lentils, green peas, enriched cereals, breads, noodles, rice, sunflower seeds, and yogurt.

When it comes to facilitating the growth of cells, producing energy, and breaking down fats, steroids, and some medications in the body, *riboflavin* (B2) is a key player. Foods rich in B2 include dairy products, eggs, lean beef and pork, organ meats (beef liver), chicken breast, salmon, fortified cereal and bread, almonds, and spinach. (B vitamins are extremely sensitive to heat, which is why unpasteurized milk typically contains larger amounts of B vitamins than pasteurized milk.)

Niacin, B3, is used by every part of the body when it comes to energy production. It also helps in creating cholesterol and fats, as well as repairing DNA. Some of niacin's effects are also known to be antioxidative. You can easily find niacin in red meat such as beef, beef liver, and pork, poultry, fish, brown rice, fortified cereals and breads, nuts, seeds, legumes, and bananas.

Pantothenic acid, or B5, focuses on breaking down fats and carbohydrates for energy. It is also critical in the production and formation of red blood cells and some sex hormones. It is found in organ meats (liver, kidney), beef, chicken breast, mushrooms, avocado, nuts, seeds, dairy milk, yogurt, potatoes, eggs, brown rice, oats, and broccoli.

Pyridoxal phosphate, otherwise known as B6, has several important functions. It assists more than a hundred enzymes in the body in breaking down proteins, carbohydrates, and fats. B6 also helps regulate homocysteine levels (high levels of this amino acid can create heart problems) and support immune and brain health. You can easily obtain B6 from meat, fish, poultry, legumes, tofu and other soy products, potatoes, and noncitric fruits such as bananas and watermelons.

Biotin (B7) is a vitamin many people have heard of because of its advertised benefits for hair, skin, and nails. The research on biotin supplementation is unfortunately inconclusive with regard to its advertised benefits.[104] Biochemically, biotin is involved in the mitochondria energy production and is, in fact, needed for healthy bones, skin, and hair. Dietary sources of biotin include beef liver, eggs (cooked), salmon, avocados, pork, sweet potatoes, nuts, and seeds.

---

[104] *Journal of Drugs in Dermatology*, "The Infatuation With Biotin Supplementation: Is There Truth Behind Its Rising Popularity?" last modified 2017.

Unlike biotin, there is one B vitamin that can actually provide more benefit to the body in its supplement form as opposed to dietary consumption: vitamin B9. The natural form of B9 is *folate*; however, *folic acid*, which is the supplement form of B9, is more easily absorbed than the folate found in food. You may have heard of the massive health benefits of folic acid for pregnant women and developing fetuses. Folic acid helps facilitate the development of the neural tube, the early formation of the brain and spine. Folic acid is also elemental in the formation of new cells. This is one reason why pregnant women should increase their folic acid consumption. Folic acid, like B6, helps lower homocysteine levels within the body, reducing the chances of developing Alzheimer's and cardiovascular disease. Although supplementation of folic acid is encouraged, you can still obtain vitamin B9 through the following food items: dark-green leafy vegetables (turnip greens, spinach, romaine lettuce, asparagus, brussels sprouts, broccoli), beans, peanuts, sunflower seeds, fresh fruits, fruit juices, whole grains, liver, seafood, and eggs. It should be noted that individuals who struggle with alcoholism may actually have a *deficiency* of folate, given that alcohol both speeds up the rate at which folate is broken down inside the body and interferes with folate absorption. People living with digestive disorders (celiac disease, IBS) also struggle to absorb adequate levels of folate.

The last vitamin we are going to highlight here is vitamin B12, otherwise known as *cobalamin*. This B vitamin helps reduce homocysteine levels, promotes the creation of new cells, is protective of neurons, and helps create red blood cells and DNA. Unfortunately for non-meat eaters, B12 is primarily obtained from animal sources, such as fish, shellfish, liver, red meat, eggs, and poultry, as well as dairy products such as milk, cheese, and yogurt. Supplementation with B12 is appropriate for those who do not consume meat, for they run the risk of being dangerously low, especially pregnant women. A developing fetus requires B12 for a healthy nervous system. Outside of diet, an all-too-common cause of vitamin B12 deficiency revolves around stomach acid, which helps the absorption of B12 into the body. Older individuals may have less stomach acid, and anyone on digestive medications that suppress stomach acid for conditions such as gastroesophageal reflux disease (GERD) or peptic ulcer disease (antacids) runs the risk of B12 deficiencies.[105]

When we think of food as fuel for our cells, we cannot help but make much more intentional decisions about what we put in our body. Whether it's to fortify the cellular membranes protecting our cells or strengthen the mitochondria inside the cell for vital energy production, what we eat helps us directly counteract the trauma we are all exposed to on a daily basis.

The final aspect of cellular health that is worth focusing on is the part of our cells that controls every aspect of who we are. Inside each cell is the nucleus, a small and separate compartment that is responsible for controlling the entire cell—how it replicates, grows, and dies. It stores the most personal intimate information we have: our DNA, the vital blueprint for how our body is uniquely made. Unfortunately, DNA is susceptible to trauma from the environment, such as excessive UV light or pesticide exposure, tobacco use (including vaping), or the way we cook or smoke certain meats.

---

[105] *National Center for Biotechnology Information (NCBI)*, "Vitamin B12 Deficiency," accessed December 22, 2024.

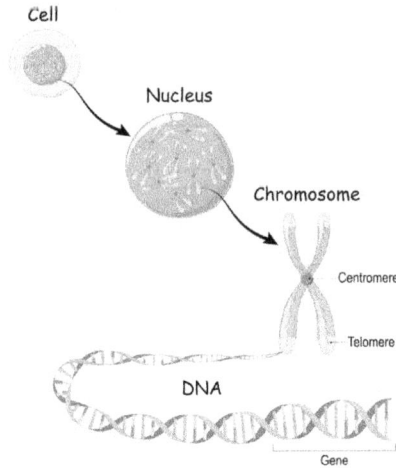

The nucleus is the control center of the cell,
safely housing DNA—the genetic blueprint that
directs all growth, repair, and function.

The ultimate objective of any living organism is to deliver its genetic material intact and unaltered, and every single cell in your body depends on this. Alterations or damage to your cellular DNA can lead to diseases of all sorts. DNA never leaves the nucleus, and because of this, it must be protected at all costs. Thankfully, the nucleus has a protective double layer called the *nuclear membrane*, also referred to as the *nuclear envelope*. This phospholipid shell keeps out large molecules while allowing in smaller ones such as oxygen and glycerol.

The nuclear membrane can be supported nutritionally in many ways similar to those that support the larger membrane of the entire cell. Healthy fats and proteins are still very much relevant here; however, the DNA faces very specific dangers. Cells and their organelles create chemical processes all day long. It's how they create proteins, send molecules to other cells, move around, grow, eat, and expel waste. All of these actions create chemical molecules, some of which, such as *free radicals*, do significant damage to the cell and its DNA. Free radicals are unstable molecules containing oxygen that react with the cell and its DNA to create destructive forces within.

It is unfortunate that many of these free radicals are naturally occurring products of normal cell functioning. Any time fats, proteins, and carbohydrates are combined with oxygen in the body to produce energy, they make free radicals. Some immune system functions also create free radicals, as do certain exercises. Remember our conversation about stress and how trauma of any kind may cause the physical breakdown of the body? Environmental stressors such as tobacco smoke, ultraviolet rays, and air pollution also cause the body to create free radicals! Of course, every aspect of the cell is susceptible to free radical damage, but consider the consequences of damaging the nucleus, the protector of your DNA. When the nucleotides that make up the spiraling staircase that is our DNA are damaged, the cell begins to make mistakes. Impaired cellular function, cell loss, or the transformation of healthy cells to cancers can occur. Programmed cell death (*apoptosis*) can spiral out of control, or uncontrolled cellular growth can happen.

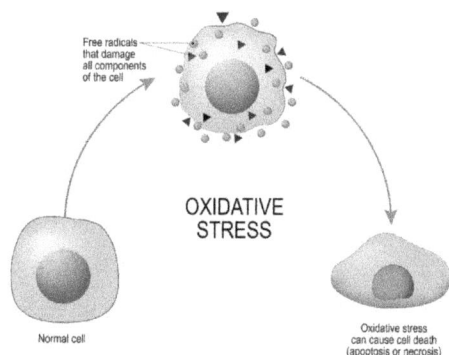

Free radicals that damage all components of the cell

OXIDATIVE STRESS

Normal cell

Oxidative stress can cause cell death (apoptosis or necrosis)

Oxidative damage is like rust eating away at your DNA, weakening the blueprint of life and setting the stage for disease and premature aging.

Free radicals, sometimes classified as *reactive oxygen species*, are being closely studied in health science now and are recognized by most scientists to be the origin of the human aging process and degenerative diseases such as cancer, autoimmune disease, and Alzheimer's disease.[106] Free radicals keep accumulating in and around us. A holistic-minded individual would see environmental stressors, such as free radicals, and see an opportunity to manage this cellular breakdown through the foods we consume. Attacking this critical issue in our society would require asking oneself, "How can I slow down the process of nucleic breakdown and DNA mutation?"

Focusing on antioxidant-rich foods is one essential piece of this puzzle. The term *antioxidant* is more appropriately discussed as a chemical property used to describe any compound that neutralizes and counteracts the damage done to cells by a free radical than to describe food. Our bodies certainly produce small quantities of antioxidants on their own. However, this is not enough to counteract the excessive amounts of cellular breakdown that occur in our bodies every day. Luckily, the foods we *choose* to consume can be a rich source of antioxidants. Vitamin C, vitamin E, and carotenoids are well-known antioxidants.

Ascorbic acid, or vitamin C, is water soluble, making it easily available to cells. It has immense immune protective qualities and is a strong antioxidant player. But vitamin C is not just an effective remedy for the sniffles; it is essential in the formation of a protein called *collagen*. Vitamin C is directly used by the following body systems: immune, nervous, circula-

---

106   Annwyne Houldsworth, "Role of Oxidative Stress in Neurodegenerative Disorders: A Review of Reactive Oxygen Species and Prevention by Antioxidants," *Brain Communications* 6, no. 1 (2024): fcad356.

tory, muscular, skeletal, and others. Because vitamin C is not held on to long, we must consume it daily for the cells and tissue to benefit. Excellent sources of vitamin C include kale, broccoli, brussels sprouts, oranges, lemons, papaya, strawberries, grapefruit, bell peppers, sweet potatoes, and tomatoes.

Another powerful antioxidant is vitamin E, *a fat-soluble* vitamin. Primarily found in plant-based oils and nuts and some fruits and vegetables, vitamin E plays a pivotal role in immune function. Nutritional sources of vitamin E include sunflower seeds, almonds, peanuts and peanut butter, pumpkin, spinach, beets, asparagus, and avocados.

Have you ever wondered why some foods have such bright hues of orange, yellow, and red? Carotenoids are the plant pigments responsible for the vibrant colors, and they too are powerful antioxidants. Carotenoids are a class of phytochemicals (or phytonutrients) and are the precursors to vitamin A, an essential vitamin for the production of white blood cells, vision, and endothelial lining. Foods that are high in carotenoids include beets, broccoli, carrots, bell peppers, mangoes, turnips, oranges, peaches, pumpkin, sweet potatoes, winter squash, spinach, and apricots.

These short lists should make one thing extremely clear: plants are key. There are significant differences between the chemical compositions of a plant that grew in the ground and a supplement that was compounded in a laboratory. Take vitamin E, for example. There are eight naturally occurring forms of vitamin E, whereas vitamin E supplementation focuses on only one form of E, *alpha-tocopherol*. Most of the research on antioxidant supplements, while still ongoing, shows that the human body benefits the most from plant-derived antioxidants (food). Nutritionists and academics believe that the phytochemicals of plants facilitate a greater antioxidative effect, and obtaining vitamins and minerals through a balanced diet is critical. Fresh fruits and vegetables and clean organic meats are essential for supplying the body with what it truly needs. Remember, B vitamins are water-soluble: they are not easily stored in the body, and any excess is expelled through the urinary tract. Taking high doses of B vitamins once a month (when you remember to) is not as beneficial as incorporating healthy food items into each meal of the day.

What we consume is critical. We live in a world of cardio-vascular disease, cancer, and premature death—all of which have been linked to high amounts of oxidative trauma. It is essential to have a balanced diet on a daily basis. Our bodies, our organs, and our cells are under daily stress. We are on track for early death and disease if we think we can choose to eat clean, healthy foods only one day a week to offset the other six days when we eat pretty much whatever strikes our fancy. That is not managing stress. In 2017, the *International Journal of Epidemiology* published a meta-analysis of ninety-five different studies analyzing cardiovascular disease, strokes, cancers, and premature deaths. The authors of this gigantic study concluded, "Fruit and vegetable intakes were associated with reduced risk of cardiovascular disease, cancer and all-cause mortality."[107]

Let's step away from the microscopes and cell slides. How many times have you been instructed on the critical importance of nutrition in the setting of a hospital, urgent care, or general

---

[107] Dagfinn Aune et al., "Fruit and Vegetable Intake and the Risk of Cardiovascular Disease, Total Cancer and All-Cause Mortality–A Systematic Review and Dose-Response Meta-Analysis of Prospective Studies," *International Journal of Epidemiology* 46, no. 3 (2017): 1029–1056.

physician's visit? How many diagnoses have you received in your life that have been accompanied by an appropriate dietary regimen? How many "wellness" visits have your children had that have included a careful analysis of what they consume all day long? Have you ever been told that the Food Guide Pyramid is dangerous to your child's health? Do you think maybe you have been left behind in the world of nutritional education?

But it may not be your medical doctor's fault. Medical schools historically have placed an extremely low priority on nutrition. In many ways, the medical-school curriculum still resembles the one taught in the early '20s, after the Flexner Report. Our understanding of nutrition has skyrocketed exponentially these past hundred years. So we must ask: If the patient's well-being truly comes first, why haven't medical schools evolved their education process? A 2015 report in the *Journal of Biomedical Education* stated that only 29 percent of US medical schools offer their med students the recommended twenty-five hours of nutrition education. The national average is 19.6 hours of nutrition education, which comes out to be less than 1 percent of the total lecture hours for a medical student.[108] To make matters worse, most of these nutrition hours are not focused on practical nutrition counseling for patients; instead, students are mainly taught complex biochemical pathways that are important to know about but are of little use when it comes to counseling everyday patients and helping them navigate complicated nutritional decisions. It's likely that many doctors would receive a failing grade on practical nutritional knowledge. A 2016 study featured in the *International*

---

[108]   Kelly M. Adams, W. Scott Butsch, and Martin Kohlmeier, "The State of Nutrition Education at US Medical Schools," *Journal of Biomedical Education* 2015 (2015): Article ID 357627.

Journal of Adolescent Medicine and Health analyzed the basic nutritional knowledge of fourth-year medical-school graduates who were entering into a pediatric residency. Alarmingly, they found that only 52 percent could answer the basic nutrition surveys correctly.[109]

Now, it could be argued that every educational program has its faults, and postgraduates of all trades can continue their learning *throughout* their career. But given the amount of time medical physicians in the United States have with each patient, things don't look promising. The average patient visit in the US is only twenty minutes, and MDs are expected to perform an incredibly long list of duties within each visit. Getting into a nuanced, sensitive conversation around nutrition may be asking too much.[110]

Why are we not seeing a greater rate of medical referrals to nutritionists and naturopaths? These are holistic doctors, who are highly educated within the realm of diet and nutrition and have the time to spend carefully with each patient. If patient care were the first priority, wouldn't medical doctors be happy and eager to refer to these health care professionals? We know too much about the importance of nutrition to condone this kind of nutritionally deficient medical practice. We see how the chemical building blocks of our food can help us manage daily stressors, treat specific signs and symptoms, and even prevent disease processes from happening.

[109]   M. Castillo et al., "Basic Nutrition Knowledge of Recent Medical Graduates Entering a Pediatric Residency Program," *International Journal of Adolescent Medicine and Health* 28, no. 4 (2016): 357–361.

[110]   Margaret Ray and John Rizzo, "Physician Incentives and Treatment Choices in Heart Attack Management," *Health Economics* 18, no. 6 (2009): 739–754.

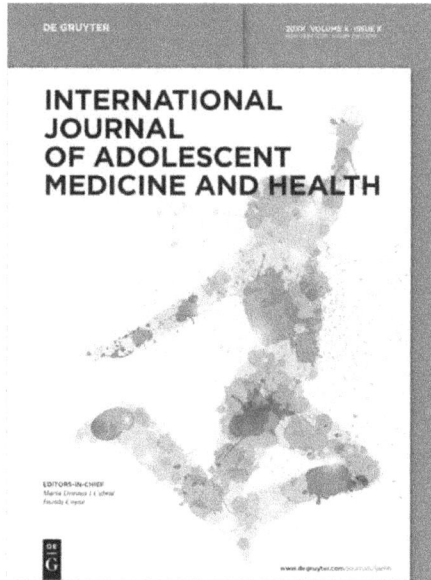

Even well-respected medical journals around the world are highlighting how today's medical students are lacking adequate training in nutrition.

Reclaiming our health through holistic healing means recognizing the fact that we are in the driver's seat during this journey. Taking ownership of our health can start only after an adequate understanding of nutrition. You can help your children understand this. You don't have to wait for *The Muppets* to create a new public service announcement or for nutrition to start trending on Instagram. We can't necessarily change our genetic framework or choose a brand-new environment to live in, but we can choose a *holistic lifestyle* that is congruent with vitality. None of this means that to be a holistically oriented human you must ignore symptoms or let conditions go untreated. There are incredibly effective and accessible resources to holistically manage one's specific symptoms and illnesses, such as naturopathic care.

CHAPTER 12

BREAKING UP
THE MONOPOLY

"You never change things by fighting the existing reality.
To change something, build a new model that makes the
existing model obsolete."

—R. Buckminster Fuller

THE EDUCATION FOR naturopathic medicine is very similar
to medical school. Naturopathic doctors study the same
basic sciences. They are required to attend extensive four-year
postgraduate programs and must pass national and state licensing exams. They are trained in primary care medicine (with
an emphasis on natural medicine), and they use traditional
Western medicine as the basis of diagnosis and treatment methods. What sets naturopathic doctors apart from their medical
colleagues is their emphasis on *natural healing* techniques, focusing on disease prevention and health promotion. Common
treatment methods used by naturopathic doctors include:

- Botanical medicine
- Clinical nutrition

- Homeopathy
- Lifestyle counseling
- Physical therapies
- Pharmacology
- IV therapy
- Minor surgery

As with the chiropractic profession, six key principles continue to be an elemental aspect of naturopathic medicine. In 1989, the six principles of naturopathic medicine were formally systematized and adopted unanimously by the American Association of Naturopathic Physicians. These principles help guide the education process of holistic providers, their diagnosis strategies, and decisions about the use of specific treatments. The first four principles—*vis medicatrix naturae, tolle causam, primum non nocere*, and *docere*—come from a long tradition of medical and philosophical thought, rooted in both naturopathic medicine and broader historical concepts of health care. These principles were often expressed in Latin to reflect their deep roots and universality. The fifth principle ("Treat the Whole Person") and the sixth principle ("Prevention"), while essential to naturopathic practice, were articulated more recently in English and likely lacked Latin counterparts at the time of formalization.

1. **The Healing Power of Nature (*Vis medicatrix naturae*)**

   Naturopathic medicine recognizes the body's inherent ability to heal itself. Doctors of naturopathic medicine work to remove barriers to this healing process. This core philosophical principle of naturopathic medicine describes the biological, bioenergetic, and physiological healing process within natural systems.

2. **Identify and Treat the Causes (*Tolle causam*)**
   Naturopathic doctors understand that the mere suppression of symptoms isn't adequate. To truly heal, we must go after the root cause of illness or disease.

3. **First Do No Harm (*Primum non nocere*)**
   Naturopathic medicine follows three principles to avoid harming the patient:
   Use methods and medicinal substances that minimize the risk of harmful side effects.
   Avoid, when possible, the harmful suppression of symptoms.
   Acknowledge and respect the individual's healing process, using the least force necessary to diagnose and treat illness.

4. **Doctor as Teacher (*Docere*)**
   Naturopathic doctors educate the patient and encourage self-responsibility for health. They also acknowledge the therapeutic value inherent in the doctor-patient relationship.

5. **Treat the Whole Person**
   Naturopathic doctors take the time to understand the unique physical, mental, emotional, genetic, environmental, and social factors that contribute to each person's state of health. This allows naturopathic doctors to tailor individual treatment protocols.

6. **Prevention**
   Naturopathic physicians emphasize disease prevention and assess risk factors and hereditary susceptibility to disease when making appropriate interventions to prevent illness. Within the holistic health paradigm, it is still important to address immediate needs

and symptoms to help patients out of their health crises. Treating someone's symptoms is not inherently an allopathic intervention. It is, however, allopathic if the suppression of that patient's condition or symptom is the point at which the naturopathic doctor and patient part ways. Thankfully, the naturopathic profession has extensive models on the healing process and contains specific guidelines on what kinds of intervention to use and why.

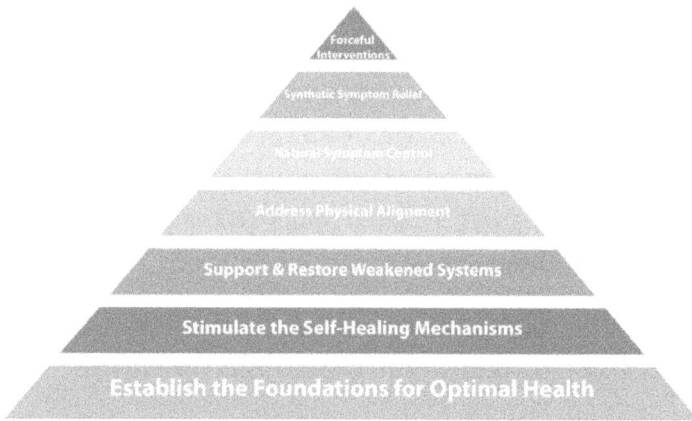

These guidelines, titled "The Therapeutic Order of Naturopathic Medicine," lay the framework for naturopathic doctors to resolve the patient's symptoms while also addressing the underlying causes.[111] The ordering of these guidelines reinforces the very first principle of naturopathic medicine, *vis medicatrix naturae*, by specifically focusing on the determinants of health.

---

[111]   Jared L. Zeff et al., "A Hierarchy of Healing: The Therapeutic Order. A Unifying Theory of Naturopathic Medicine," in *Textbook of Natural Medicine*, ed. Joseph E. Pizzorno and Michael T. Murray (Missouri: Churchill Livingstone, 2013).

Dr. Jared Zeff, ND, Lac—current president and founder of the Institute for Advanced Studies in the Healing Arts in Portland, Oregon, and founder of the Naturopathic Cancer Conference—published this groundbreaking framework for naturopathic care in the early 1990s. However, this early framework contained only four items. It wasn't until his collaboration with Dr. Pamela Snider in 1998 that the remaining three were added. This therapeutic order, in holding true to the philosophy, works from the least invasive methods of treatment to the most invasive. Intervention starts at the first level with the inside healing properties of the individual. Note that this order is not rigid, not "cookie cutter." It should be tailored specifically to each person. Though treatment may start in general, it gradually becomes more and more specific and targeted. The following summarizes the seven components and stages of The Therapeutic Order of Naturopathic Medicine.

Level One—Establish the Conditions for Health

There are several *determinants of health* that massively affect the health (or illness) of an individual: inborn, behavioral, social, cultural, environmental, and spiritual. These determinants, according to the naturopathic field, are the soil or terrain in which health or illness arise. Level One places the most emphasis on the *patient's responsibility for his or her health*. Whether it be strengthening our own inborn factors, removing the factors that disturb our health, or establishing factors that promote it, we must be actively involved in this stage.

Level Two—Stimulate the Healing Power of Nature and Self-Healing Processes

Once the determinants of health are identified and obstacles to healing removed, naturopathic physicians apply general stimulation to engage the global healing response, or self-healing. This starts with *vis medicatrix naturae*. The body heals itself, and the physician can help produce the right circumstance. The approaches of homeopathy, needling, hydrotherapy, and physical medicine are all examples of how NDs aim to stimulate the self-healing response without adding anything of substance.

Level Three—Support and Restore Weakened Systems

In some cases, the weakened or damaged body system (or organ) requires more than just stimulation to improve. Whether the system or organ is weak or damaged, blocked or congested, or overactive and irritated, naturopathic doctors use a broad scope of healing practices to bring restoration and repair. Examples of interventions are botanical medicine, endocrine balancing, professional-grade supplements, homeopathy, counseling, manual therapies, and acupuncture.

Level Four—Correct Structural Integrity

Problems with our structure inevitably arise from stress, and they create stress on our internal system. Simple therapies include spinal manipulation, therapeutic massage, acupressure, and Rolfing and other forms of hands-on therapy. Therapeutic movement, biomechanical rehab, and physical therapy may all be used to help improve structure. Naturopaths recognize structural issues to be a symptom of a larger problem. According to the published therapeutic order, NDs expect structural corrections to be required "only occasionally and for the results to be more or less permanent, if the underlying organic disturbance is corrected."

A note regarding spinal manipulation: An important distinction between a chiropractic *adjustment* and spinal *manipulation* can be based on both the intent and measurement of the outcome. A chiropractic adjustment focuses on the location of subluxated segments (neurological interference) in the spine and the removal of that neurological interference via the high velocity, low amplitude force of the adjustment. Competent chiropractors will also use various objective measurements to determine the neurological effect that took place (e.g., thermal scanning, computerized range of motion, leg-length changes, surface electromyography, heart rate variability). An *adjustment* to the nervous system can occur with or without that "cracking" sound. A *manipulation*, on the other hand, is often performed when there is joint fixation causing pain or other soft tissue impairments. The emphasis on primary causes versus secondary compensation, neurological effects, and specific techniques is not used in most spinal-manipulation cases.

Level Five—Addressing Pathology through Natural Means

When a patient moves through the first four levels of this therapeutic order, that patient tends to get better, which of course makes sense when you consider that almost every human is living with some sort of barrier to optimal health.

Remembering that the body is a self-healing organism helps one understand why most people heal with minimal, specific intervention. However, there are times when it is necessary to address a patient's specific pathology or symptoms head-on. It shouldn't be a surprise to see that the naturopathic order uses *natural* methods of symptom management before moving on.

Level Six—Addressing Pathology through Pharmaceuticals or Synthetics

Using plants or other botanicals as a method of symptom management is a *low force* intervention. Usually, such interventions carry far fewer side effects and physiologically work with the biochemical pathways inside the body. Pharmaceutical drugs and other synthetic medicines work more specifically with their interaction and are more directive of the body's biochemical pathways. For these reasons, in addition to the higher rate of adverse effects, these methods are *high force* interventions.

Level Seven—Suppress or Surgically Remove Pathology

Sometimes people are so far down the path of illness and injury that they require immediate suppression of their symptoms, even if this temporarily ignores the causation of their illness. Holistic doctors of all kinds recognize the important role conventional medical doctors play in the healing journey. Where holistic providers, such as naturopaths and chiropractors, go the extra mile is their emphasis on the causative factors. By suppressing the pathology or symptom, it's not unusual for the patient to *feel* better, even as his or her underlying problem gets worse and worse. This kind of intervention is the last step in the therapeutic order.

These seven steps have been explored, refined, and codified through a series of publications, faculty retreats, discussions, and meetings. This therapeutic order has created the guidelines for thousands of skilled and compassionate doctors to deliver incredible healing changes for people around the world. Allopathic (mainstream) medicine has been able to attach the label of *alternative* to many different forms of health care, and this label often carries with it a negative undertone.

A recent study conducted by the Australian Research Center in Complementary and Integrative Medicine examined the state of naturopathic care on an international scale.[112] This research has helped illuminate just how mainstream naturopathic care is and the breadth of its practice. Currently there are ninety-eight countries where naturopathic doctors are practicing, with most of those doctors in North America, where regulatory positions are the most established. Thirty European countries (Europe is the birthplace of naturopathy) have naturopaths practicing, as do 43 percent of countries in Latin America. Throughout Asia, naturopathic physicians are sought out. In Australia and New Zealand, many consider them to be primary and conventional. The study analyzed over eight hundred patient visits in naturopathic clinics in fourteen different countries. A majority of patients in these clinics were female, and most had chronic health conditions. These patients had, for the most part, at least one follow-up visit. Their most

---

[112]   Amie Steel et al., "Overview of International Naturopathic Practice and Patient Characteristics: Results from a Cross-Sectional Study in 14 Countries," *BMC Complementary Medicine and Therapies* 20, no. 1 (2020): 59.

common categories of health conditions were musculoskeletal, gastrointestinal, and mental health challenges. A significant number of patient visits were also categorized as "general wellness." As the researchers pointed out, every year, naturopaths see patients of all ages for a variety of health concerns. They use evidence-based intervention such as nutrition and lifestyle changes, through the lens of the therapeutic order.

When it comes to the treatment methods used, most naturopaths incorporate dietary changes, lifestyle behavioral changes, herbal medicines, and nutritional supplementation. Despite the attempts to diminish the efficacy of naturopaths, it remains true that countless patients facing a variety of health challenges have been helped by these methods. Take blood pressure, for instance. You may know several people struggling to gain control of their blood pressure, perhaps even yourself. Nearly one out of two adults in the United States battle with hypertension (high blood pressure).

BLOOD PRESSURE CATEGORY	SYSTOLIC mm Hg (upper number)	DIASTOLIC mm Hg (lower number)
NORMAL	LESS THAN 120	LESS THAN 80
ELEVATED	120–129	LESS THAN 80
HIGH BLOOD PRESSURE (HYPERTENSION) STAGE 1	or 130–139	80–89
HIGH BLOOD PRESSURE (HYPERTENSION) STAGE 2	140 OR HIGHER or	90 OR HIGHER

*

Many people find lasting relief from blood pressure issues through naturopathic care, which supports the body's natural balance with lifestyle changes, nutrition, and targeted herbal or mineral support.

Currently, the American Heart Association's consensus for *healthy* blood pressure is less than 120/80. The top number represents *systolic* blood pressure—the force produced by the heart pumping blood out to the body. The bottom number is *diastolic* blood pressure—the pressure inside of the blood vessels *between* each heartbeat.

- *Elevated* blood pressure ranges between 120–129 (systolic) and less than 80 (diastolic).
- *Hypertension Stage 1* ranges from 130 to139 over 80 to 89.
- *Hypertension Stage 2* is 140+ over 90 and above.

Bastyr University, specializing in natural medicine and science in Washington State, studied the relationship between naturopathic care and blood pressure changes. Their medical center, Bastyr Center, received more than 34,000 patient visits in 2022. Hypertensive patients receiving care in this clinic between 2001 and 2006 were studied. Naturopathic doctors were aiming to observe the changes in both systolic blood pressure and diastolic blood pressure over time, as well as how many patients could achieve control of their blood pressure—with *control* being any measurement less than 140/90. The researchers at Bastyr categorized their hypertensive patients using a different system from what the AHA used. In this study, the following coding system was used:

- Stage 1 Hypertension: 140–159 over 90–99
- Stage 2 Hypertension: 160+ over 100+

These high blood pressure ratings should be taken extremely seriously. Patients with uncontrolled hypertension have *double the risk* for cardiovascular mortality compared with those who have normal, healthy blood pressure. The characteristics of the naturopathic care in this study are summarized below:[113]

- On average, the patients in this study received 8.7 doctor visits for their concerns.
- Average timespan of care was 13.8 months.
- 97 percent of patients received *dietary counseling* that was reemphasized at each visit. Tobacco and alcohol use also ranked high in discussion topics.
- 68.2 percent received counseling to increase *physical activity*.
- For 76 percent of patients, ND care remained mostly adjunctive.
- 23.5 percent of patients use ND care as primary care.

The figure below was taken from the actual study, showing the different clinical recommendations made to patients, the physiological reasoning behind them, and the frequency with which they were given.

---

[113] Richard Bradley et al., "Observed Changes in Risk during Naturopathic Treatment of Hypertension," *Evidence-Based Complementary and Alternative Medicine* 2011 (2011): Article ID 826751.

Dietary change (97.6%) =
↓ inflammation and
Na-induced fluid retention

Physical activity (68.2%) =
↑ flow mediated dilation and
↓ resting heart rate

Omega-3 fatty acids (55.3%) =
↑ cell membrane function and
↓ inflammation

Rauwolfia (50.6%) =
↓ sympathetic tone

Magnesium (43.5%) =
↑ smooth muscle relaxation

CoQ10 (38.8%) =
↑ myocardial ATP

Haw-thorne
(32.9%) =
↑ AOX and O_2
use

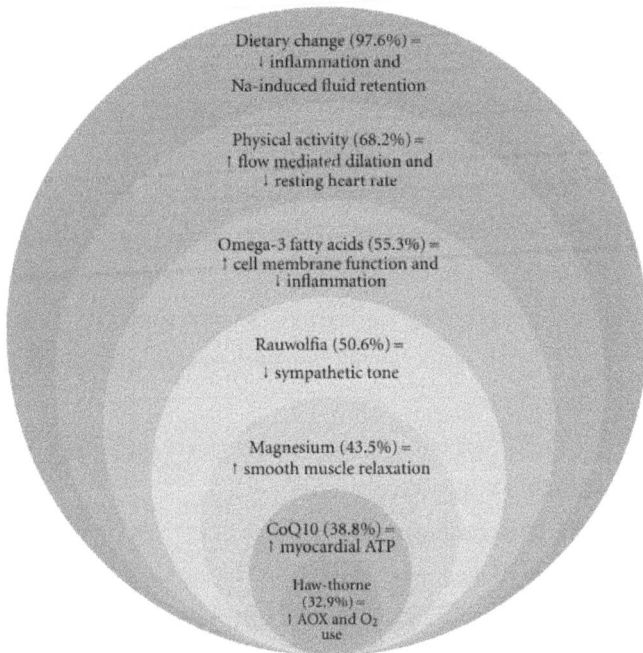

Figure 1: Hypothetical model for select elements of naturopathic treatment of hypertension. Values in parentheses indicate the percentage of patients receiving this recommendation. Citations for the hypothetical actions are included in the main text. AOX, antioxidant action; ATP, adenosine triphosphate; Na, sodium; O_2, oxygen.

The results of this study, published in 2011, show promising outcomes for those struggling with extreme hypertension.[114] The participants averaged sixty-one years of age, and 51 percent of participants had systolic blood pressure over 160 and diastolic blood pressure over 100, even though 47 percent of individuals in this group were already on antihypertensive

---

[114]   Richard Bradley et al., "Observed Changes in Risk during Naturopathic Treatment of Hypertension," *Evidence-Based Complementary and Alternative Medicine* 2011 (2011): Article ID 826751.

medication prescribed by their medical doctor. Patients in both Stage 1 and 2 hypertension (as defined by the authors of this study) saw a reduction in their overall blood pressure. Patients with Stage 2 hypertension saw, on average, a 26mmHg reduction of systolic blood pressure as well as an 11mmHg reduction of diastolic pressure. *Before* the start of naturopathic intervention, only 14 percent of the patients were in the group that was considered to have "controlled" blood pressure (less than 140 over less than 90). *After* naturopathic care, 44 percent of the group was considered to have control.

As positive as these results are for patients struggling with severe blood pressure issues, these findings represent just a single study. What do clinical outcomes look like when we broaden our scope? Despite that naturopathic care is classified as *alternative* throughout the health care world, research into the breadth and scope of naturopathic treatment is hardly scarce.

In 2019, researchers and physicians—led by Dr. Stephen Myers and Vanessa Vigar at the National Centre for Naturopathic Medicine in Australia—published the current state of naturopathic research evidence on *whole system, multimodality naturopathic medicine*. The authors of this study only included cases in which a naturopath was the treating doctor. Thirty-three studies across seven countries were included, assessing the health changes in over nine thousand patients. Conditions such as cardiovascular disease, chronic musculoskeletal pain, type 2 diabetes, polycystic ovarian syndrome, anxiety, and depression were all included. A requirement for inclusion was that each study had to have a minimum of five case studies. The data collected on patient outcomes for these various conditions and naturopathic care were promising.

Below are the results of this study, published in *The Journal of Alternative and Complementary Medicine.*[115]

Cardiovascular Disease

Myers and Vigar included nine studies investigating the outcomes for patients with current cardiovascular disease (CVD) or the development of CVD risk factors (such as hypertension). Two of the studies included were randomized control trials, and three studies included multicomponent care. The authors concluded, "Overall, these studies show naturopathic treatment results in a clinically significant benefit for treatment of hypertension, reduction in metabolic syndrome parameters, and improved cardiac outcomes post-surgery."

Type 2 Diabetes

Four studies were included in this category, two prospective and two retrospective. Three of these studies originated from Bastyr University and were focused on blood glucose management. The fourth study came from India, studying inpatient care for type 2 diabetes. The results of these studies showed that "naturopathic treatment results in a significant benefit for treatment of diabetes, with reductions in HbA1c that are clinically relevant."

---

[115]   Stephen P. Myers et al., "The State of the Evidence for Whole-System, Multi-Modality Naturopathic Medicine: A Systematic Scoping Review," *The Journal of Alternative and Complementary Medicine* 25, no. 2 (2019): 141–168.

Musculoskeletal Pain

Six studies were included for this category. Clinical conditions included chronic back pain, rotator cuff tendinitis, multiple sclerosis, temporomandibular disorder, and generalized chronic body pain. Four of these studies were randomized control trials. Myers and Vigar concluded, "Overall, this diverse group of studies shows that naturopathic treatment decreased pain scores to a degree comparable or better than standard care or other active treatment controls." What is the significance of a randomized control trial (RCT)? RCTs are often praised for being the gold standard of a research trial, for they provide the most reliable evidence with the lowest levels of bias when it comes to understanding the effectiveness of an intervention.

Mood Disorders

Four studies were included to evaluate the effectiveness of naturopathic treatment for mood disorders, one of which was an RCT. Also included was a single study for both anxiety and depression, and a single study on bipolar disorder. The authors concluded, "Significant reductions in anxiety and depression levels were shown across this group of studies."

CHAPTER 13

WHAT DOES IT MATTER?

"For the meaning of life differs from man to man, from day to day, and from hour to hour. What matters, therefore, is not the meaning of life in general but rather the specific meaning of a person's life at a given moment."

—Viktor Frankl

WHAT DOES A lifetime of memories with your loved ones feel like? Recall the feeling of holding your newborn child for the first time, proposing to your life partner, sunsets on a beach with your friends, and being there for your family in tough times. Can these emotions even be accurately described? When I ponder the meaning of a life well spent, built on human connection, I can't help but think of two people in my own life, my grandmother and my niece. They live on the same property, a beautiful, decent-sized plot of land in western Washington, with green fields, apple trees, white fences, a rustic red barn, chickens, and horses. Despite that my grandmother, Joyce, is in her eighties, she is still very much tending to her farm as she did back in the '90s when she purchased it. Gardening is her passion year-round. Mowing, weeding, chopping firewood, and up until recently, bucking hay bales were all part of her daily and weekly routine. Safe to say, sitting down and knitting were not Joyce's thing.

A few yards down live my sister and her family, including, at this writing, baby Maisie—a happy, giggly, and all-too-curious toddler. Joyce and Maisie spend an incredible amount of time together. With plenty of acres and animals to keep Maisie's curiosity satisfied, Joyce allows my sister and brother-in-law to focus on their professions and other commitments. Joyce doesn't mind all this responsibility; in fact, she *loves* her role as great-grandmother—with a total of four great-grandkids all of whom she sees on a daily basis.

When I think about the exceptional relationship Joyce and Maisie have, I can't help but get emotional. How rare is that level of connection in our world today? Go to your local mall and watch grandparents and grandchildren together. You will be lucky to find a group not separated by an iPhone or tablet. How often do we call our grandparents outside of holidays and birthdays? Are we as connected with our loved ones today as we were when we were younger? We have an entire generation of children being raised with no connection to the world of sixty or seventy years ago. Think about the seniors in your life. Do they have quality conversations on a regular basis? Are they given the opportunity to provide and contribute, as so many of them wish to do? Or are they isolated like, sadly, millions of senior citizens in this country?

My grandmother is an incredible human. Joyce is strong, both physically and mentally. She has never had a major surgery. She manages her blood sugar almost exclusively through nutrition and exercise. Joyce provides for multiple members of her family, is independent, and is a true leader in our family. She is a clear example of health. My little niece, Maisie, is developing at an outstanding rate. She is meeting her milestones on time. She is bright and engaged. She has a sense of humor. She has never been bottle-fed. Maisie was born in water, had her spine evaluated and adjusted for vertebral subluxation within a day of being born, and has never needed medication. She spends time outside every day and gets to be barefoot in the grass. Maisie has minimal screen time, eats whole organic foods, and has healthy bonds with all members of her family. She too is a clear example of health and well-being.

This is the "sense of coherence" that all humans need to answer the key question raised by Aaron Antonovsky: "What makes a person healthy?" Antonovsky spent his life creating academic frameworks to chase this question, which led to the creation of salutogenesis.

In order to have complete coherence within our lives, we must first be able to *comprehend* the problems we face. And really, that could mean anything—comprehending the stressors we face each day on a physical level, an emotional level, and chemically. Do we comprehend how these traumas affect our bodies? Furthermore, do we understand the signs and symptoms we are experiencing? Do we have holistically centered doctors in our lives helping us make sense of our blood work, our X-rays, and our problems?

It's not that healthy people live free from aches and pains and conditions. Healthy individuals move through life with the understanding of how their body works in relationship to their environment. They understand that you cannot eat the way the Food Pyramid recommends and expect to have normal blood pressure and blood sugar. They understand that even with the absence of any symptoms, they may still have aspects of their health to repair and strengthen. Healthy people understand that every cell operates in unison and every organ system is interrelated, and they know how to manage their problems. Recognizing that nutritional habits can be either life-enhancing or life-ending, holistic individuals go out of their way to cut certain items out altogether (trans fats, processed foods, vegetable oils). They also go out of their way to eat a balanced, whole food, organic diet to support entire bodily function rather than simply satiating hunger by any means necessary.

A holistic-minded person understands the power of the nervous system and its control over every cell, tissue, and organ. They understand that if there's a breakdown in neural communication, a breakdown in bodily function ensues. Life is naturally stressful—physically, mentally, and chemically—and this is why millions of people now use chiropractic as a part of their regular health care routine, as it was designed to be over a hundred years ago.

And finally, a holistic individual does not ignore signs and symptoms. Such a person understands that health is not always easy to maintain, and we do develop conditions and diseases. It's a part of the human experience, sadly. However, rather than throwing medications at the problem to mask the symptoms, this individual seeks out holistic doctors such as naturopaths to help them address specific symptoms from the inside out—through much gentler and safer methods.

These are all ways healthy people manage themselves in a stressful, chaotic world. But Aaron Antonovsky knew there was one more crucial concept to establish: *meaningfulness*—something so few people have in their life. What may seem like a small idea is actually everything. It guides every single thought, action, behavior, and outcome. The meaning we attach to our circumstances changes how we behave. We can see that entirely evident in the way our society has become so dependent on medicine and allopathic health care. Perhaps the lack of attachment people have to true health is one reason why the medical establishment has been so successful.

The next time you are in front of a group of people, ask them this very simple question: "Who here wants to live to be one hundred?" At one time, you could ask that question, and everyone would have gladly raised their hand. Nowadays, fewer and fewer people would answer that way. Why? You might hear responses like, "I don't want to be on a lot of medications." Or "I don't want to be a burden to my kids." Or, sadly, "What's the point?" The *meaning* we have in our lives is everything. What would it look like in your life to have more time with your loved ones? What would it feel like to have less fear around health care debt? What would it be like to have your parents around for the birth of your children and to see your children create lifelong memories with the grandparents? Do you want your children to grow up without the need for medications and surgery? The answers to these questions are the guiding light for how you navigate through the world of health care. Don't be so quick to dismiss them.

This is not a book about the meaning of life. For those important existential questions, I leave it to the experts—the Dalai Lama, Jesus Christ, Thich Nhat Hanh, Yoda, or the guru of your choice. This book is about *root causes*—the root cause of our medical dependency and all the adverse effects in our society that this dependency has caused. If these archaic paradigms and systems brought to us by mainstream Westernized medicine have led to disastrous states of health and disease, then perhaps the root cause of health lies in a different approach to health care. Living our lives with a salutogenic view of the world may be the key. It would certainly explain what's happening inside of Blue Zones.

Author, producer, and award-winning journalist Dan Buettner has long been fixated on longevity. He has traveled the world in search of the common denominators of health, well-being, and living to an advanced age—the *root causes*, if you will, of what it takes to live to be one hundred without drugs, surgeries, and disability. Throughout his explorations into longevity, Dan has teamed up with the National Institute on Aging and *National Geographic* to answer some of the most pressing questions of our lives. If you've never heard of the Blue Zones Project nor seen the popular TED Talk on it, it clearly highlights the importance of living a vitalistic, dynamic life. Through the use of epidemiological data, statistics, birth certificates, and other research methodology, Dan and his team were able to identify five specific geographical regions where individuals were living to be up to and over one hundred years old, at an astonishing rate of ten times greater than the United States. Loma Linda, California; Nicoya, Costa Rica; Sardinia, Italy; Ikaria, Greece; and Okinawa, Japan all have extraordinary numbers of vital men and women living well into their late nineties and to one hundred. The results for these specific regions—Blue Zones—are not coincidences. Each of these zones contains specific lifestyle patterns that are conducive to living to be one hundred years of age and remaining happy and content.

Within each of these Blue Zones can be found the following shared characteristics:

- Naturally occurring daily movement.
- A sense of purpose.
- Built-in routines to combat stress.
- Eating in moderation—with larger proportions of plants in each meal.
- Regular (but moderate) alcohol consumption with friends.
- Belonging to some kind of faith-based community.
- Family-first focus, and a tight-knit group of friends.

These are what successful centenarians are doing around the world. Recall how the World Health Organization defined health: "A state of complete physical, mental and social well-being and not merely the absence of disease or infirmity." Each of these habits of these men and women, living in Blue Zones, hit on one of these aspects of physical strength, mental resiliency, and social well-being. Of course, illness and disease exist in these geographic zones. It's not that there are zero occurrences of sickness. It's that the *holistic lifestyles* of these men and women are much better suited to handle signs and symptoms.

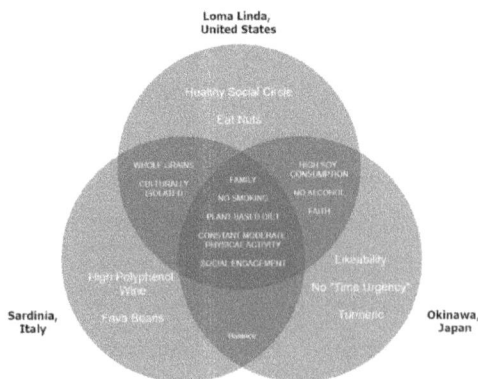

Loma Linda,
United States

Healthy Social Circle

Eat Nuts

WHOLE GRAINS

HIGH SOY
CONSUMPTION

CONTINUALLY
EVOLVED?

FAMILY

NO SMOKING

NO ALCOHOL

PLANT-BASED DIET

FAITH

CONSTANT MODERATE
PHYSICAL ACTIVITY

SOCIAL ENGAGEMENT

High Polyphenol
Wine

Likeability

No "Time Urgency"

Sardinia,
Italy

Fava Beans

Turmeric

Okinawa,
Japan

Humor

Blue Zones teach us that longevity isn't about one
secret—it's the result of a whole lifestyle built on purpose,
connection, movement, and nourishing food.

Think about a day in the life of someone who lives in Okinawa and upholds traditional Japanese practices. Many if not most meals in Okinawa involve sitting on the ground, including tea-time and general workspaces. It's not uncommon for an elderly Okinawan to stand up from the floor or squat down and sit hundreds of times a day. This may not seem like a physically laborious task such as going to the gym or joining a running club, but the amount of physical work it takes to sit and squat all day long is lifesaving, especially the more one ages. Strengthening the muscles around the hips and in the legs provides more stability and balance, decreasing the risk of falling. Regular use of our lower extremities vastly improves blood circulation to the brain. And sitting upright on the floor is one of the best ways to preserve spinal health, including vertebral discs.

It's not uncommon for Okinawans to have personal gardens. Of course, spending an increased amount of time outside on a regular basis is a positive influence on our health. But consider the mental and social benefit it can have for a senior citizen—having a job or task, having something to take pride in, sharing with others, and a sense of purpose and contribution. Apart from being a fun hobby in this culture, gardens also provide food. Over 50 percent of the traditional Okinawan diet is vegetable-based. And being on an island, men and women here have easy and regular access to omega-3 rich sources of protein from the sea.

Aside from physical conditioning and clean-eating practices, one of the most spectacular aspects of Okinawan culture revolves around their *support networks*. Referred to as *moai*, this ritual is intended to bring secure social connections to all members of the moai. Some of these social bonds are formed by children as young as five, and they often last an entire lifetime. Members provide support, whether emotional or financial, regularly engage in social outings, check in on each other daily, and provide one another with a great sense of comfort. Okinawa has healthy habits present in every aspect of their daily culture. Living a holistic life and having remarkable outcomes is not just a privilege of the rich and famous. It is available for all those born in this region.

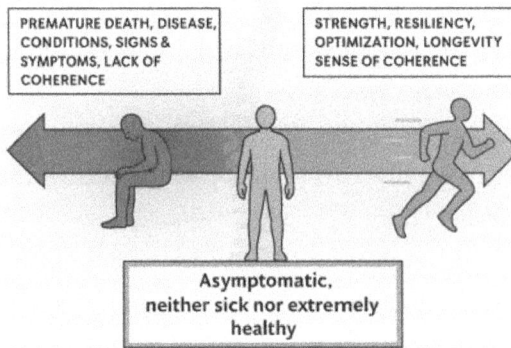

PREMATURE DEATH, DISEASE, CONDITIONS, SIGNS & SYMPTOMS, LACK OF COHERENCE

STRENGTH, RESILIENCY, OPTIMIZATION, LONGEVITY SENSE OF COHERENCE

Asymptomatic, neither sick nor extremely healthy

Health exists on a spectrum—not just sick or well—where true wellness means moving beyond being symptom-free toward strength, resilience, and optimized living.

If health and well-being exist on a spectrum, then we have easily identified those living on the extreme end of vitality, thriving, and improving. We know of places where chronic illness is minimal, health care expenditures are within normal limits, medical debt doesn't cripple families, and doctors and nurses aren't leaving the profession in record numbers. In these places, people naturally live to be one hundred plus with their friends, continuing to support their families and create meaningful bonds.

During the Blue Zones project, one centenarian in Japan was interviewed about her family life. When asked about how it felt to be able to be present in their lives, she described the feeling of holding her great-great-great-grandchild as "jumping into heaven." Contrast the life of a one-hundred-year-old Okinawan with that of any average senior citizen living in America. In the United States, it is not abnormal to live alone in a semi-isolated state, in which lifestyles across all ages are largely sedentary. You can probably picture your grandparent's favorite recliner positioned in front of the television. There are, unfortunately, too many examples in which the lifestyles of the elderly in America differ from those in any of the Blue Zones across the globe. How many of our grandparents, aunts, uncles, or parents are living on the other end of the health spectrum—where chronic illness is running rampant, medical debt is soaring, and medications and surgery are regular events? How many amazing people in the United States live with crippling fear of one bad fall or insurance deciding to stop covering their medication? How many of our loved ones are living life without purpose or connections, with zero sense of coherence in their lives?

And now we have arrived at *you*. Is there any sense of coherence in the life you're living? Do the stressors you encounter stack up until you inevitably become sick or injured several times a year? Are you able to comprehend what these traumas even are, what they do to you, and what the symptoms you have really mean? Has it felt like with each passing year it becomes harder and harder to stay on top of your health? Do you manage your health on a regular basis through a holistic, whole-body means, or just when emergencies arise?

What does your health mean to you? Are you concerned about not being there for those you love with all your heart? Not being present in the life around you? If you feel like you're at a pivotal moment in your life, a crossroads—good. Use the emotions that came up in response to any of these questions to your benefit. Remember, the rider of the elephant can only do so much without the elephant's buy-in. It's okay to allow emotions to guide us if we keep our destination in mind. Millions of men and women, children and the elderly, have these questions and emotions. Whether they know it or not, their health shapes the way they do everything. This is where most of our health care efforts should be made—those living in the middle of this health and wellness spectrum, those who sway back and forth, inching closer and closer to illness and injury each year.

If you wish to live a truly holistic life, focus on what keeps you and your children *healthy* rather than on sickness alone. It's no longer an option to sit on your hands and wait for outdated governmental and medical practices to change. We must be our own advocates.

We can no longer wait until our habits and lifestyles "catch up to us." That isn't living a holistic lifestyle. Procrastination is perhaps the largest thief of well-being. The lifestyle habits we practice every single hour of every single day can be holistic and honoring of our health. Or the exact opposite—pulling us deeper and deeper into poor health. We can help ourselves, our children, our family, and our friends get on the right path toward a long and meaningful life.

It's okay to seek help for health concerns. Not seeking the care your body needs and refusing to see a doctor or physician isn't holistic either. Doctors of chiropractic and naturopathy, nutritionists, counselors, trainers—all are here to help guide you through your unique health needs, help you heal through crises, and even help prevent them from happening in the first place. The vision I hold for humanity is like Joyce and Maisie's story. I wish all children born into the world today can grow up surrounded by the wisdom and guidance that only grand-parents and great-grandparents can instill, in which social and emotional attention is given freely, in which motor skills and cognition can be stimulated naturally in a safe environment. I wish more children could live more normal lives, and not the "new normal" that has been slowly redefined for them, in which screen time influences their neurological development, in which it's normal to need antibiotics regularly, and where social interaction isn't prioritized.

I wish that all of the elderly in our society could have a meaningful life rich with friendships and purpose that get them out of bed every day. May they live in a world where medication and surgery doesn't loom over them like a large cloud. May they get to save their money—instead of spending it on lifelong prescription medication use. Instead, may they spend it freely on what makes them *happy*. Our elderly men and women need to know that even if they catch a bacteria or virus, they are strong enough to handle it and can live with peace of mind—rather than the *anxiety* that is so much a part of the lives of too many senior citizens.

I wish that everyone between the ages of one and one hundred can live comfortably, knowing they can influence their life for the better—by focusing on what they can directly control: their habits, their belief systems, and their lifestyles. I wish that, even in the face of great turmoil in our world, we do not have to wait until everything gets fixed for us to start to live just a little bit healthier each day.

Within every single outcome in your life lies a root cause. Don't stop asking yourself questions such as "Why is that?" or "How can that be?" Start discovering the reasons why you're sick, why you're unfulfilled, and why—no matter what—you just can't seem to break the mold you're stuck in.

Don't just settle with weeding out the outdated health beliefs and practices you've picked up along the way; it's our responsibility to cultivate that which is healthy and good in this garden of life we are creating. Whether it be for yourself here and now or for the generations to come whom you'll never meet, the root causes of a healthier, more connected, and free society start with the seeds we plant today.

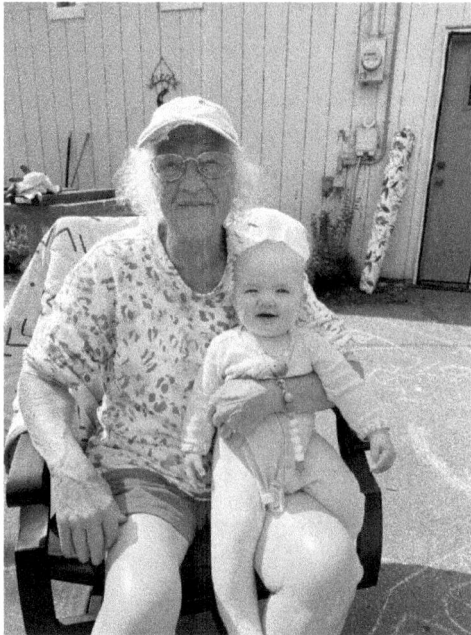

Joyce with her fourth great-grandchild, Maisie.

BIBLIOGRAPHY

Introduction

Toyota Industries Corporation. "Toyoda Sakichi | History | Company | Toyota Industries Corporation." Toyota Industries Corporation. Accessed April 3, 2023. https://www.toyota-industries.com/company/history/toyoda_sakichi/.

Ohno, Taiichi. *Toyota Production System: Beyond Large-Scale Production.* 1st ed. Portland, OR: Productivity Press, 1988. https://Doi.org/10.4324/9780429273018.

McNeill, Jeff. "Sakichi Toyoda and the Five Whys Root Cause Analysis." Jeff McNeill. Last modified October 31, 2015. Accessed April 3, 2023. https://jeffmcneill.com/sakichi-toyoda-and-the-five-whys-root-cause-analysis/.

Schwartz, Aaron L., Bruce E. Landon, Adam G. Elshaug, Michael E. Chernew, and J. Michael McWilliams. "Measuring Low-Value Care in Medicare." *JAMA Internal Medicine* 174, no. 7 (2014): 1067-1076. doi:10.1001/jamainternmed.2014.1541.

Osborn, Robin, David Squires, and Michelle M. Doty. "Paying for Prescription Drugs Around the World: Why Is the U.S. an Outlier?" The Commonwealth Fund. Last modified October 16, 2017. Accessed April 3, 2023. https://www.commonwealth-fund.org/publications/issue-briefs/2017/oct/paying-prescrip-tion-drugs-around-world-why-us-outlier?redirect_source=/publications/issue-briefs/2017/oct/prescription-drug-costs-us-outlier#6.

"Chronic Disease Prevention and Health Promotion." Centers for Disease Control and Prevention. Accessed April 3, 2023. https://www.cdc.gov/chronicdisease/index.htm.

"Heart Disease and Stroke Prevention: Factsheet." Centers for Disease Control and Prevention. Accessed April 3, 2023. https://www.cdc.gov/chronicdisease/resources/publications/factsheets/heart-disease-stroke.htm.

"Coronary Artery Disease (CAD)." Mayo Clinic. Accessed April 3, 2023. https://www.mayoclinic.org/diseases-con-ditions/coronary-artery-disease/symptoms-causes/syc-20350613#:~:text=Coronary%20artery%20disease%2C%20also%20called,are%20almost%20always%20to%20blame.

Katz, Mitchell H., and Vinay Prasad. "The Surprising History of the "NNT"." *JAMA Internal Medicine* 171, no. 13 (2011): 1272-1274. doi:10.1001/archinternmed.2011.300.

Stergiopoulos, Nikolas J., and David L. Brown. "Initial Coro-nary Stent Implantation with Medical Therapy vs Medical Therapy Alone for Stable Coronary Artery Disease: Meta-Analysis of Randomized Controlled Trials." *Archives of Internal*

Medicine 172, no. 4 (2012): 312–319. https://doi.org/10.1001/archinternmed.2011.1484.

Medscape. *Medscape Lifestyle Report 2017: Race and Ethnicity, Bias and Burnout.* Accessed December 22, 2024. https://www.medscape.com/features/slideshow/lifestyle/2017/overview.

Shanafelt TD, Boone S, Tan L, et al. Burnout and satisfaction with work-life balance among US physicians relative to the general US population. Arch Intern Med. 2012;172:1377–1385. doi:10.1001/archinternmed.2012.3199.

Department for Professional Employees, AFL-CIO. "Safe Staffing Critical for Patients and Nurses." Department for Professional Employees, AFL-CIO. https://www.dpeaflcio.org/factsheets/safe-staffing-critical-for-patients-and-nurses#_edn33. Accessed April 3, 2023.

Aiken, L. H., Clarke, S. P., Sloane, D. M., Sochalski, J., & Silber, J. H. (2002). Hospital Nurse Staffing and Patient Mortality, Nurse Burnout, and Job Dissatisfaction. *JAMA*, 288(16), 1987–1993. doi:10.1001/jama.288.16.1987

Aiken, Linda H., et al. "Nurses' reports on hospital care in five countries." Health Affairs 20, no. 3 (2001): 43-53.

IsHak W, Nikravesh R, Lederer S, Perry R, Ogunyemi D, Bernstein C. Burnout in medical students: a systematic review. Clin Teach. 2013;10:242–245.Frajerman, Alexandre, Morvan.

Yann, Krebs Marie-Odile, Gorwood Philip, and Chaumette Boris. "Burnout in medical students before residency: a systematic review and meta-analysis." Eur Psychiatry 55 (2019): 36-42.

Chapter 1

Standing Bear, Luther. *Land of the Spotted Eagle.* Lincoln and London: University of Nebraska Press.

Hodge, Frederick Webb. Medicine Men & Healing Practices. Washington, DC: The Smithsonian Institution, 1906.

Underhill, Ruth M. "The Medicine-Man of the American Indian and his Cultural Background." *Nature* 138 (1936): 268. doi:10.1038/138268b0.

Linderman, Frank B. *Pretty-Shield: Medicine Woman of the Crows.* HarperCollins, 2021.

Deloria Jr., Vine. *The World We Used to Live In: Remembering the Powers of the Medicine Men.* Fulcrum Publishing, 2006, pp. xxv-xxvi.

Deloria Jr., Vine. *The World We Used to Live In: Remembering the Powers of the Medicine Men.* Fulcrum Publishing, 2006, p. 84.

Parker, Steve. *A Short History of Medicine.* DK, 2019.

Dove, Mourning. Quoted in "Mourning Dove." *Encyclopedia of World Biography*, 2nd ed., vol. 9, Gale, 2004, p. 222.

LaFargue, Michael. *The Tao of the Tao Te Ching: A Translation and Commentary*. Albany: State University of New York Press, 1992.

Yutang, Lin. *The Wisdom of Laotse*. New York: Modern Library, 1948.

Unschuld, Paul U., Hermann Tessenow, and Zheng Jinsheng. "Front Matter." In *Huang Di Nei Jing Su Wen: An Annotated Translation of Huang Di's Inner Classic – Basic Questions: 2 Volumes*, 1st ed., 1-4. University of California Press, 2011.

Parker, Steve. *A Short History of Medicine*. DK, 2019.

Shabrawy, C. 1992. Interview with Naguib Mahfouz.

Joshua J. Mark. "Egyptian Medicine." *Encyclopedia Britannica*. https://www.worldhistory.org/Egyptian_Medicine/#google_vignette.

Rogers, Kara. *Medicine and Healers Through History*. New York: The Rosen Publishing Group, Inc., 2011.

The Papyrus Ebers. Translated by Cyrill Phillips Bryan, with an introduction by Professor Grafton Elliot Smith. London: ARES PUBLISHERS INC, 1930.

Queijo, J. (2010). Breakthrough!: How the 10 greatest discoveries in medicine saved millions and changed our view of the world. FT Press Science.

North, Michael. *Greek Medicine: The Hippocratic Oath*. U.S. National Library of Medicine, 2002. Accessed October 22,

2023. https://www.nlm.nih.gov/hmd/topics/greek-medicine/index.html#case1.

Tountas, Y. (2009). The historical origins of the basic concepts of Health Promotion and education: The role of ancient Greek philosophy and medicine. *Health Promotion International*, *24*(2), 185–192. https://doi.org/10.1093/heapro/dap006.

Chapter 2

Michel de Montaigne: The complete essays. (1993). Penguin Books.

Rosenberg, Charles E. *The Care of Strangers: The Rise of America's Hospital System*. Baltimore: Johns Hopkins University Press, 1987.

Georgetown University Health Policy Institute, "Prescription Drugs" https://hpi.georgetown.edu/rxdrugs/ (accessed July 30, 2023).

"Museum of Osteopathic Medicine at A.T. Still University," https://www.atsu.edu/museum-of-osteopathic-medicine/museum-at-still (accessed July 30, 2023).

General William Tecumseh Sherman, speech to the graduating class of the Michigan Military Academy, June 19, 1879.

Gevitz, Norman. "Center or Periphery? The Future of Osteopathic Principles and Practices." *J Am Osteopath Assoc*, 2006, 106(3), 121-129.

Keating, Joseph C., Carl S. Cleveland, and Michael Menke. *Chiropractic History: A Primer.* Association for the History of Chiropractic, 2004.

The Chiropractic 1897 (Jan); Number 17 (Palmer College Archives).

Snider, P., & Zeff, J. "Unifying Principles of Naturopathic Medicine: Origins and Definitions." *Integrative Medicine (Encinitas)* 18, no. 4 (2019): 36-39. PMID: 32549831.

Donohue, Julie. "A History of Drug Advertising: The Evolving Roles of Consumers and Consumer Protection." *The Milbank Quarterly* 84, no. 4 (2006): 659–699. https://doi.org/10.1111/j.1468-0009.2006.00464.x.

Chapter 3

Duffy, Thomas P. 2011. "The Flexner Report--100 Years Later." *The Yale Journal of Biology and Medicine* 84 (3): 269–276.

Baer, Hans A. "The Sociopolitical Status of U.S. Naturopathy at the Dawn of the 21st Century." *Medical Anthropology Quarterly* 15 (2001): 329-346. doi:10.1525/maq.2001.15.3.329.

Report of the Task Force on Medicaid and Related Programs. United States: U.S. Department of Health, Education, and Welfare, 1970.

Chapter 4

American Institute of Homeopathy. "History of AIH: Our Heritage, Our Future." Accessed December 22, 2024. https://homeopathyusa.org/history-of-aih-our-heritage-our-future/.

Zebroski, Bob. *A brief history of pharmacy: Humanity's search for Wellness.* Routledge, 2015.

Boyer, Paul S. The oxford companion to united states history. Oxford etc.: Oxford University Press, 2004.

Ober, K.P. "The pre-Flexnerian reports: Mark Twain's criticism of medicine in the United States." *Annals of Internal Medicine* 126, no. 2 (1997): 157-163. doi:10.7326/0003-4819-126-2-199701150-00012.

Silver, Shawn A. "Thanks, But No Thanks: How Denial of Osteopathic Service in World War I and World War II Shaped the Profession" *Journal of Osteopathic Medicine* 112, no. 2 (2012): 93-97. https://doi.org/10.7556/jaoa.2012.112.2.93.

The Journal of the American Osteopathic Association. 1940. "Did the association fail its country?" Vol. 40, no. 3: 153.

Johnson, Claire D., and Bart N. Green. "Looking Back at the Lawsuit That Transformed the Chiropractic Profession Part 4: Committee on Quackery." *Journal of Chiropractic Education* 35, no. S1 (2021): 55–73.

Green, Bart N., and Claire D. Johnson. "Fighting Injustice: A Historical Review of the National Chiropractic Antitrust Committee." *Journal of Chiropractic Humanities* 26 (2019): 19–30.

Chapter 5

Penn Nursing. "History of Hospitals." Nursing History and Healthcare, University of Pennsylvania School of Nursing. Accessed December 22, 2024. https://www.nursing.upenn.edu/nhhc/nurses-institutions-caring/history-of-hospitals/.

Rowland, Darrel. "75 Years Ago, a Landmark Bill for American Hospitals." *Ohio Capital Journal*, August 19, 2021. https://ohiocapitaljournal.com/2021/08/19/75-years-ago-a-landmark-bill-for-american-hospitals/.

U.S. Social Security Administration. "Historical Background and Development of Social Security." Accessed December 22, 2024. https://www.ssa.gov/history/aja1265.html.

U.S. Social Security Administration. "Title XVIII of the Social Security Act: Health Insurance for the Aged and Disabled." Accessed December 22, 2024. https://www.ssa.gov/OP_Home/ssact/title18/1800.htm.

Burns, David M. "Cigarette Smoking Behavior in the United States." *Tobacco Control* 4, suppl. 1 (1995): S2–S8. Accessed December 22, 2024. https://tobaccocontrol.bmj.com/content/4/Suppl_1/S2.

Carolina Demography. "Mortality and Cause of Death, 1900 vs. 2010." Accessed December 22, 2024. https://carolinademography.cpc.unc.edu/2014/06/16/mortality-and-cause-of-death-1900-v-2010/.

Centers for Disease Control and Prevention. "About Chronic Diseases." Last reviewed February 7, 2023. Accessed December

22, 2024. https://www.cdc.gov/chronic-disease/about/index.
html.

National Cancer Institute. "Cancer Statistics." Accessed December 22, 2024. https://www.cancer.gov/about-cancer/understanding/statistics.

Centers for Disease Control and Prevention. "National Diabetes Statistics Report." Last reviewed June 29, 2022. Accessed December 22, 2024. https://www.cdc.gov/diabetes/communication-resources/diabetes-statistics.html.

Fullman, Nancy, Emilie J. Heidari, Hunter York, et al. "Measuring Performance on the Healthcare Access and Quality Index for 195 Countries and Territories and Selected Subnational Locations: A Systematic Analysis from the Global Burden of Disease Study 2016." *The Lancet* 391, no. 10136 (2018): 2236–2271. Accessed December 22, 2024. https://www.thelancet.com/journals/lancet/article/PIIS0140-6736(18)30994-2/fulltext.

Peterson-KFF Health System Tracker. "How Do Mortality Rates in the U.S. Compare to Other Countries?" Last updated May 19, 2022. Accessed December 22, 2024. https://www.healthsystemtracker.org/chart-collection/mortality-rates-u-s-compare-countries/.

Advisory Board. "Maternal Mortality Rates: The U.S. vs. Other Developed Nations." Last updated June 5, 2024. Accessed December 22, 2024. https://www.advisory.com/daily-briefing/2024/06/05/maternal-mortality.

Stock, Sarah E., et al. "Maternal and Neonatal Outcomes Associated with Operative Vaginal Delivery Using Forceps and Vacuum: A Retrospective Cohort Study." *The BMJ* 383 (2023): e075058. https://pmc.ncbi.nlm.nih.gov/articles/ PMC10585424/.

Nolte, Ellen, and C. Martin McKee. "Measuring the Health of Nations: Updating an Earlier Analysis." *Health Affairs* 26, no. 1 (2007): 71–83.

Shimony, Hagar, L. Miller, P. Reich, N. R. Banull, M. Burch, M. Bryan, and A. María Arbeláez. "Pediatric Diabetes Mellitus Hospitalizations and COVID-19 Pandemic Response Measures." *Diabetes Research and Clinical Practice* 207 (January 2024): 111060.

Chapter 6

Guy, GP Jr., Zhang K, Bohm MK, et al. "Vital Signs: Changes in Opioid Prescribing in the United States, 2006–2015." *MMWR Morbidity and Mortality Weekly Report* 66 (2017): 697–704.

National Institute on Drug Abuse. "Overdose Death Rates." *National Institutes of Health.* Accessed February 8, 2025. https:// nida.nih.gov/research-topics/trends-statistics/overdose-death-rates.

Centers for Disease Control and Prevention. "Drug and Opioid-Involved Overdose Deaths—United States, 2013–2017." *Morbidity and Mortality Weekly Report* 67, no. 12 (2018):

1419–1427. Accessed December 22, 2024. https://www.cdc.gov/mmwr/volumes/67/wr/mm6712a1.htm.

Asfaw, Abay, Brian Quay, Tim Bushnell, and Regina Pana-Cryan. "Injuries That Happen at Work Lead to More Opioid Prescriptions and Higher Opioid Costs." *Journal of Occupational and Environmental Medicine* 64, no. 12 (December 1, 2022): e823–e832. https://doi.org/10.1097/JOM.0000000000002709.

Trecki, John. "A Perspective Regarding the Current State of the Opioid Epidemic." *JAMA Network Open* 2, no. 1 (2019): e187104. https://doi.org/10.1001/jamanetworkopen.2018.7104.

Hadland, Scott E., et al. "Physician Prescribing and Pharmaceutical Industry Marketing: Implications for Stimulant Misuse." National Institutes of Health HEAL Initiative. Last modified July 2021. Accessed December 22, 2024. https://heal.nih.gov/files/2021-07/physician-prescribing-stimulant-misuse-hadland.pdf.

Ornstein, Charles, and Ryann Grochowski Jones. "Doctors Prescribe More of a Drug If They Receive Money from a Pharma Company Tied to It." *ProPublica*, March 17, 2016. Accessed December 22, 2024. https://www.propublica.org/article/doctors-prescribe-more-of-a-drug-if-they-receive-money-from-a-pharma-company-tied-to-it.

U.S. Department of Health and Human Services, Office of the Assistant Secretary for Planning and Evaluation. *Savings Available Under Full Generic Substitution of Multiple Source Brand Drugs in Medicare Part D.* Published July 23, 2018. Ac-

cessed December 22, 2024. https://aspe.hhs.gov/sites/default/
files/migrated_legacy_files/182231/DP-Multisource-Brands-
in-Part-D.pdf.

Light, Donald W., and Joel R. Lexchin. "Pharmaceutical
Research and Development: What Do We Get for All That
Money?" *BMJ* 345 (2012): e4348. https://doi.org/10.1136/bmj.
e4348.

Gagnon, Marc-André, and Joel Lexchin. "The Cost of Pushing
Pills: A New Estimate of Pharmaceutical Promotion Expenditures in the United States." *PLoS Medicine* 5, no. 1 (2008): e1.
https://doi.org/10.1371/journal.pmed.0050001.

Hay, Michael, David W. Thomas, John L. Craighead, Celia
Economides, and Jesse Rosenthal. "Clinical Development Success Rates for Investigational Drugs." *Nature Biotechnology* 32,
no. 1 (2014): 40–51. Accessed December 22, 2024. https://
diyhpl.us/~nmz787/pdf/Clinical_development_success_rates_
for_investigational_drugs.pdf.

The Washington Post. "Analysis of Research Articles Published
in the New England Journal of Medicine." Accessed December
22, 2024. https://www.washingtonpost.com/wp-srv/special/
business/NEJM-articles/.

Ehrhardt, Stephan, Lawrence J. Appel, and Curtis L. Meinert.
"Trends in National Institutes of Health Funding for Clinical Trials Registered in ClinicalTrials.gov." *JAMA* 314, no. 23
(2015): 2566–2567. https://doi.org/10.1001/jama.2015.12206.

Drugwatch. "Big Pharma & Clinical Trials: Funding, Influence & Corruption." Accessed December 22, 2024. https://www.drugwatch.com/featured/clinical-trials-and-hidden-data/.

Jefferson, Tom, Mark A. Jones, Peter Doshi, Chris B. Del Mar, Carl J. Heneghan, Igho J. Onakpoya, and Matthew J. Thompson. "Neuraminidase Inhibitors for Preventing and Treating Influenza in Adults and Children." *Cochrane Database of Systematic Reviews* 2014, no. 4 (2014): CD008965. https://doi.org/10.1002/14651858.CD008965.pub4.

Abramson, John. *Sickening: How Big Pharma Broke American Health Care and How We Can Repair It.* Boston: Mariner Books, 2022.

Bombardier, Claire, Loren Laine, Arthur Burgos-Vargas, Bruce Davis, Richard Day, Michael Ferraz, Christine J. Hawkey, et al. "Comparison of Upper Gastrointestinal Toxicity of Rofecoxib and Naproxen in Patients with Rheumatoid Arthritis." *The New England Journal of Medicine* 343, no. 21 (2000): 1520–1528. https://doi.org/10.1056/NEJM200011233432103.

Abramson, John. Interview by Joe Rogan. *The Joe Rogan Experience.* Episode 1756. Spotify, January 12, 2022. https://open.spotify.com/episode/xyz123.

CBS News. "Timeline of Vioxx-Related Events." Accessed December 22, 2024. https://www.cbsnews.com/news/timeline-of-vioxx-related-events/.

UNC School of Medicine. "Medicine Grand Rounds: Dr. John Abramson Presents 'Why We Can't Trust the Evidence in Evidence-Based Medicine'." Accessed December 22, 2024. https://www.med.unc.edu/medicine/event/medicine-grand-rounds-dr-john-abramson-presents-why-we-cant-trust-the-evidence-in-evidence-based-medicine/.

Corporate Crime Reporter. "John Abramson on How Big Pharma Broke American Health Care." Accessed December 22, 2024. https://www.corporatecrimereporter.com/news/200/john-abramson-on-how-big-pharma-broke-american-health-care/.

AlphaSense. *Medtech and Medical Device Outlook for 2024 & Beyond.* Accessed December 22, 2024. https://www.alpha-sense.com.

U.S. Food and Drug Administration. *510(k) Premarket Notification Program: Guidance for Industry and FDA Staff.* Accessed December 22, 2024. https://www.fda.gov/media/82395/download.

Somberg, Matthew D., Harmeeth S. Sandhu, Javad Parvizi, and Peter B. Mears. "Analysis of FDA-Approved Orthopaedic Devices and Their Recalls." *The Journal of Bone & Joint Surgery* 98, no. 6 (2016): 517–524. Accessed December 22, 2024. https://journals.lww.com/jbjsjournal/Abstract/2016/03160/Analysis_of_FDA_Approved_Orthopaedic_Devices_and.12.aspx.

PR Newswire. "High-Price Device Race to Innovate: Medical Devices Fuels More Product Recalls." Last modified February

8, 2017. Accessed December 22, 2024. https://www.prnews-wire.com/news-releases/high-price-device-race-to-innovate-medical-devices-fuels-more-product-recalls-300402968.html.

Drugwatch. "FDA 510(k) Clearance Process: How Medical Devices Reach the Market." Accessed December 22, 2024. https://www.drugwatch.com/fda/510k-clearance/#:~:text=Between%2095%20and%2098%20percent,have%20received%20little%20government%20scrutiny.

Panish Shea & Boyle LLP. "510(k) Loophole in Medical Device Cases." Accessed December 22, 2024. https://www.pstriallaw.com/legal-news/510k-loophole-in-medical-device-cases.

Chapter 7

Haidt, Jonathan. *The Happiness Hypothesis: Finding Modern Truth in Ancient Wisdom.* New York: Basic Books, 2006.

BioPharma Dive. "Pharma Ad DTC Marketing: $2.8 Billion Spent on TV in 2018." Last modified October 15, 2018. Accessed December 22, 2024. https://www.biopharmadive.com/news/pharma-ad-dtc-marketing-2018-spend-TV-congress/533319/.

Vaughan, Diane. *The Challenger Launch Decision: Risky Technology, Culture, and Deviance at NASA.* Chicago: University of Chicago Press, 1996.

Cleveland Clinic Journal of Medicine. "ADHD: Diagnosis and Management in Children and Adolescents." *Cleveland Clinic*

Journal of Medicine 84, no. 11 (2017): 873–881. Accessed December 22, 2024. https://www.ccjm.org/content/84/11/873.

Chapter 8

Lindström, Bengt, and Monica Eriksson. "Contextualizing Salutogenesis and Antonovsky in Public Health Development." *Health Promotion International* 21, no. 3 (September 2006): 238–244. https://doi.org/10.1093/heapro/dal016.

Eriksson, Monica, Bengt Lindström, and Jarl A. Lilja. "A Sense of Coherence and Health: Salutogenesis in a Societal Context: Åland, a Special Case?" *Journal of Epidemiology & Community Health* 61, no. 8 (2007): 684–688. https://doi.org/10.1136/jech.2006.047498.

Antonovsky, Aaron. *Unraveling the Mystery of Health: How People Manage Stress and Stay Well.* San Francisco: Jossey-Bass Publishers, 1987.

Chapter 9

TeachMePhysiology. "Cellular Adaptations." Accessed December 22, 2024. https://teachmephysiology.com/histology/tissue-structure/cellular-adaptations/.

Merck Manual Professional. "Red Blood Cell Production." Accessed December 22, 2024. https://www.merckmanuals.com/professional/hematology-and-oncology/approach-to-the-patient-with-anemia/red-blood-cell-production.

Cleveland Clinic. "Vitamin Deficiency Anemia." Accessed December 22, 2024. https://my.clevelandclinic.org/health/diseases/17732-vitamin-deficiency-anemia.

Chapter 10

Ierano, John. "Chung-Ha Suh PhD: The Proof of Subluxation. The Final Report of Chiropractic Research at the University of Colorado, 2017." *Asia-Pacific Chiropractic Journal* 2, no. 4 (2021). Accessed December 22, 2024. https://apcj.net/papers-issue-2-4/#IeranoSuh.

Haavik, Heidi. "About Dr. Heidi Haavik." Accessed December 22, 2024. https://heidihaavik.eu/pages/about-dr-heidi-haavik.

Lelic, D., Niazi, I. K., Holt, K., Jochumsen, M., Dremstrup, K., Yielder, P., Murphy, B., Drewes, A., and Haavik, H. "Manipulation of Dysfunctional Spinal Joints Affects Sensorimotor Integration in the Prefrontal Cortex: A Brain Source Localization Study." *Neural Plasticity* 2016 (2016): Article ID 3704964.

Safer Care Victoria. *Chiropractic Spinal Manipulation of Children Under 12: Independent Review.* October 2019. Accessed December 22, 2024. https://www.safercare.vic.gov.au/sites/default/files/2019-10/20191024-Final%20Chiropractic%20Spinal%20Manipulation.pdf.

Sarnat, Richard L., James Winterstein, and Jerrilyn A. Cambron. "Clinical Utilization and Cost Outcomes from an Integrative Medicine Independent Physician Association: An Additional 3-Year Update." *Journal of Manipulative and Physiological Therapeutics* 30, no. 4 (2007): 263–269.

Chapter 11

Siri-Tarino, Patty W., Qi Sun, Frank B. Hu, and Ronald M. Krauss. "Meta-Analysis of Prospective Cohort Studies Evaluating the Association of Saturated Fat with Cardiovascular Disease." *The American Journal of Clinical Nutrition* 91, no. 3 (March 2010): 535–546. https://doi.org/10.3945/ajcn.2009.27725.

Prentice, Ross L., Barbara Caan, Rowan T. Chlebowski, Lesley Tinker, Marcia L. Stefanick, Garnet Anderson, Aaron Aragaki, et al. "Low-Fat Dietary Pattern and Risk of Invasive Breast Cancer: The Women's Health Initiative Randomized Controlled Dietary Modification Trial." *JAMA* 295, no. 6 (2006): 629–642. https://doi.org/10.1001/jama.295.6.629.

Centers for Disease Control and Prevention (CDC). "LDL and HDL Cholesterol and Triglycerides." Last modified May 17, 2021. Accessed December 22, 2024. https://www.cdc.gov/cholesterol/about/ldl-and-hdl-cholesterol-and-triglycerides.html.

American Heart Association. "Trans Fat." Accessed December 22, 2024. https://www.heart.org/en/healthy-living/healthy-eating/eat-smart/fats/trans-fat.

Light, Luise. *What to Eat: The Ten Things You Really Need to Know to Eat Well and Be Healthy.* New York: McGraw-Hill, 2006.

Microbe Notes. "Phospholipid Bilayer: Structure, Types, Properties, Functions." Accessed December 22, 2024. https://

microbenotes.com/phospholipid-bilayer-structure-types-properties-functions/.

Frontiers in Cell and Developmental Biology. "Effects of Trans Fatty Acids on Cellular Function and Membrane Integrity." Accessed December 22, 2024. https://www.frontiersin.org/journals/cell-and-developmental-biology/articles/10.3389/fcell.2019.00187/full.

Journal of Drugs in Dermatology. "The Infatuation With Biotin Supplementation: Is There Truth Behind Its Rising Popularity?" Last modified 2017. Accessed December 22, 2024. https://jddonline.com/articles/the-infatuation-with-biotin-supplementation-is-there-truth-behind-its-rising-popularity-a-comparativ-S1545961617P0496X/.

National Center for Biotechnology Information (NCBI). "Vitamin B12 Deficiency." Accessed December 22, 2024. https://www.ncbi.nlm.nih.gov/medgen/784757.

Houldsworth, Annwyne. "Role of Oxidative Stress in Neurodegenerative Disorders: A Review of Reactive Oxygen Species and Prevention by Antioxidants." *Brain Communications* 6, no. 1 (2024): fcad356. https://doi.org/10.1093/braincomms/fcad356.

Niki, E., et al. "Interaction among Vitamin C, Vitamin E, and Beta-Carotene." *The American Journal of Clinical Nutrition* 62, no. 6 (1995): 1322S–1326S. https://doi.org/10.1093/ajcn/62.6.1322S.

Aune, Dagfinn, Edward Giovannucci, Paolo Boffetta, Lars T. Fadnes, Naomi Keum, Teresa Norat, Darren C. Greenwood,

Susanna C. Larsson, Dag S. Tonstad, and Elio Riboli. "Fruit and Vegetable Intake and the Risk of Cardiovascular Disease, Total Cancer and All-Cause Mortality–A Systematic Review and Dose-Response Meta-Analysis of Prospective Studies." *International Journal of Epidemiology* 46, no. 3 (2017): 1029–1056. https://doi.org/10.1093/ije/dyw319.

Adams, Kelly M., W. Scott Butsch, and Martin Kohlmeier. "The State of Nutrition Education at US Medical Schools." *Journal of Biomedical Education* 2015 (2015): Article ID 357627. https://doi.org/10.1155/2015/357627.

Castillo, M., R. Feinstein, J. Tsang, and M. Fisher. "Basic Nutrition Knowledge of Recent Medical Graduates Entering a Pediatric Residency Program." *International Journal of Adolescent Medicine and Health* 28, no. 4 (2016): 357–361. https://doi.org/10.1515/ijamh-2015-0019.

Ray, Margaret, and John Rizzo. "Physician Incentives and Treatment Choices in Heart Attack Management." *Health Economics* 18, no. 6 (2009): 739–754. https://doi.org/10.1002/hec.1390.

Chapter 12

World Naturopathic Federation. "Naturopathic Education Comparison Table." Last modified May 2023. Accessed December 22, 2024. https://worldnaturopathicfederation.org/wp-content/uploads/2023/05/Naturopathic-education-comparison-table_final.pdf.

American Association of Naturopathic Physicians. "Blog." Accessed December 22, 2024. https://americannaturopathic.org/blog.html.

Zeff, Jared L., Pamela Snider, Stephen Myers, and Zora De-Grandpre. "A Hierarchy of Healing: The Therapeutic Order. A Unifying Theory of Naturopathic Medicine." In *Textbook of Natural Medicine*, edited by Joseph E. Pizzorno and Michael T. Murray, 2013. Missouri: Churchill Livingstone.

Steel, Amie, Hazel Foley, Robert Bradley, Jon Wardle, Hope Foley, and Jon Adams. "Overview of International Naturopathic Practice and Patient Characteristics: Results from a Cross-Sectional Study in 14 Countries." *BMC Complementary Medicine and Therapies* 20, no. 1 (2020): 59. https://doi.org/10.1186/s12906-020-2851-7.

American Heart Association. "The Facts About High Blood Pressure." Accessed December 22, 2024. https://www.heart.org/en/health-topics/high-blood-pressure/the-facts-about-high-blood-pressure.

Whelton, Paul K., Robert H. Carey, Wilbert S. Aronow, et al. "2017 ACC/AHA/AAPA/ABC/ACPM/AGS/APhA/ASH/ASPC/NMA/PCNA Guideline for the Prevention, Detection, Evaluation, and Management of High Blood Pressure in Adults: A Report of the American College of Cardiology/American Heart Association Task Force on Clinical Practice Guidelines." *Journal of the American College of Cardiology* 71, no. 19 (2018): e127–e248. https://doi.org/10.1016/j.jacc.2017.11.006.

Bradley, Richard, Editha Kozura, Jolanta Kaltunas, Erin B. Oberg, James Probstfield, and Annette L. Fitzpatrick. "Observed Changes in Risk during Naturopathic Treatment of Hypertension." *Evidence-Based Complementary and Alternative Medicine* 2011 (2011): Article ID 826751. https://doi.org/10.1093/ecam/nep219.

Myers, Stephen P., Vanessa Vigar, et al. "The State of the Evidence for Whole-System, Multi-Modality Naturopathic Medicine: A Systematic Scoping Review." *The Journal of Alternative and Complementary Medicine* 25, no. 2 (2019): 141–168. https://doi.org/10.1089/acm.2018.0340.

Chapter 13

SAGE Journal Article: Buettner, Dan. "The Blue Zones: Lessons for Living Longer from the People Who've Lived the Longest." *American Journal of Lifestyle Medicine* 10, no. 5 (2016): 318–321. https://doi.org/10.1177/1559827616637066.

Springer Article: Stenner, Kayleigh, Crystal L. MacGregor, Joseph C. Baker, and David R. Brown. "Blue Zones: Centenarian Modes of Physical Activity: A Scoping Review." *Journal of Public Health* 31, no. 2 (2022): 221–235. https://doi.org/10.1007/s12062-022-09396-0.

Blue Zones. "Moai: This Tradition Is Why Okinawan People Live Longer, Better." Last modified August 2018. Accessed December 22, 2024. https://www.bluezones.com/2018/08/moai-this-tradition-is-why-okinawan-people-live-longer-better/.

IMAGE CREDITS

https://www.mountsinai.org/health-library/discharge-in-structions/angioplasty-and-stent-heart-discharge

https://collections.library.yale.edu/catalog/2094464?utm_source=chatgpt.com

https://www.loc.gov/resource/lcnclscd.2014514432.1A002/?sp=4&st=image https://lccn.loc.gov/2014514432

https://commons.wikimedia.org/wiki/File:Portraits_of_Famous_Men_-_Yellow_Emperor_(Huangdi).jpg

Credit: Acupuncture: points controlling kidneys, Chinese. Wellcome Collection. Source: Wellcome Collection. https://creativecommons.org/licenses/by-nc/4.0/

Ebers papyrus prescription for asthma treatment.
U.S. National Library of Medicine/National Institutes of Health
https://www.britannica.com/topic/Ebers-papyrus

Source: Heka, holding two serpents crossing each other with the hind of a lion as the symbol on his head in the magical form https://commons.wikimedia.org/w/index.php?search=h eka&title=Special:MediaSearch&type=image

Rod of Asclepius https://commons.wikimedia.org/w/index. php?search=rod+of+asclepius&title=Special:MediaSearch&t ype=image

https://commons.wikimedia.org/w/index.php?search=medica l+Caduceus&title=Special:MediaSearch&type=image

https://commons.wikimedia.org/wiki/File:The_School_of_ Athens_by_Raffaello_Sanzio_da_Urbino.jpg

https://commons.wikimedia.org/wiki/File:Hippocratis_ju- siurandum.jpg

https://www.stillacademy.pl/andrew-taylor-still/

https://commons.wikimedia.org/wiki/File:Dr_A.T._Still_ and_Mrs._Annie_Morris,_his_amanuensis._Wellcome_ L0040493.jpg

Courtesy of the Palmer Archive Collections (Pending per- mission)

Advertisement for Lydia E. Pinkham's Vegetable Compound 1882 https://commons.wikimedia.org/wiki/File:Lydia_E._ Pinkham%27s_Vegetable_Compound_ad_1882.jpg

Source: Rockefeller Foundation Archive https://commons.wikimedia.org/wiki/File:Aflexner21.jpg

https://meridian.allenpress.com/jce/article/35/S1/25/470445/ Looking-back-at-the-lawsuit-that-transformed-the

https://meridian.allenpress.com/jce/article/35/S1/45/470440/
Looking-back-at-the-lawsuit-that-transformed-the

Committee on Quackery Minutes 1964-1974. Chicago, IL:
American Medical Association; 1964–1974.
Taken from: https://meridian.allenpress.com/jce/article/35/
S1/55/470442/Looking-back-at-the-lawsuit-that-trans-
formed-the

The 4 chiropractors (plaintiffs), from left to right: Michael
Pedigo, James Bryden, Chester Wilk, and Patricia Arthur.
https://meridian.allenpress.com/jce/article/35/S1/85/470441/
Looking-back-at-the-lawsuit-that-transformed-the

Getzendanner S. Permanent injunction order against AMA.
JAMA. 1988; 259 (1): 81– 82. https://meridian.allenpress.
com/jce/article/35/S1/97/470436/Looking-back-at-the-law-
suit-that-transformed-the

Newsies at Skeeter's Branch. They were all smoking. St.
Louis, Missouri. 1910. Taken from: https://rarehistorical-
photos.com/child-laborers-newsboys-1910/

Aaron Antonovsky, the father of Salutogenesis
Taken from: https://alchetron.com/Aaron-Antonovsky

https://www.ncbi.nlm.nih.gov/books/NBK435812/figure/
ch11.Fig3/

https://commons.wikimedia.org/wiki/File:Brain-diagram-
pink-6289600.svg

https://commons.wikimedia.org/wiki/File:1206_The_Neu-
ron.jpg

https://commons.wikimedia.org/wiki/File:Brain_stem_
parts.png

https://commons.wikimedia.org/wiki/File:Foramen_mag-
num_-_superior_view_-_animation.gif

https://commons.wikimedia.org/wiki/File:Cervical_Spine_
Cross_View.png

https://commons.wikimedia.org/wiki/File:Pain_and_plea-
sure_(1917)_(14596881008).jpg

iStock

https://onlinelibrary.wiley.com/doi/10.1155/2016/3704964

https://commons.m.wikimedia.org/w/index.php?search=lipid
+bilayer&title=Special:MediaSearch&type=image

https://commons.wikimedia.org/wiki/File:Blue_Zone_Re-
search_Adaptation.png

Images marked with an asterisk (*) were created by the author using AI-assisted design software.

ABOUT THE AUTHOR

D R. Avery R. Champagne is the owner and clinical director of Radiant Health Chiropractic in Lacey, Washington. His practice focuses on supporting patients with chronic health challenges and children with neurodevelopmental delays through a holistic and individualized approach. He earned his Doctor of Chiropractic degree with honors from Life Chiropractic College West in the Bay Area of California, becoming the youngest graduate in his class. During his studies, he developed a deep passion for prenatal and pediatric chiropractic care, furthering his expertise through training with the International Chiropractic Pediatric Association (ICPA). He lives in Washington, where he enjoys the natural beauty of the Pacific Northwest.

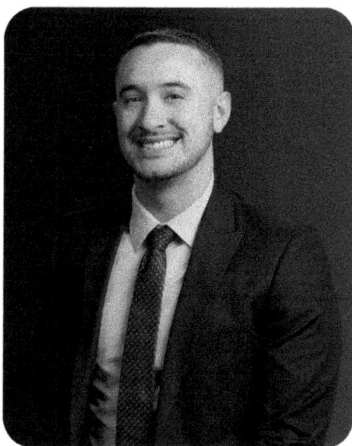